HOW TO HEAL DRY SKIN NATURALLY

THE 20 BEST DRY SKIN HOME REMEDIES

KINNARI ASHAR

Illustrated by
NEIL GERMIO

WARNINGS AND DISCLAIMERS

CONTENTS

THANKS FOR YOUR PURCHASE

Get Your Next SF Nonfiction Book FREE!

Claim the book of your choice at:

www.SFNonfictionBooks.com/Free-Book

You will also be among the first to know of all the latest releases, discount offers, bonus content, and more.

Go to:

www.SFNonfictionBooks.com/Free-Book

Thanks again for your support.

INTRODUCTION

There's so much to love about the fall season, from the breezy chill in the air to the gorgeous leaves changing colors to the first pumpkin spice latte.

But the cold, crisp air can wreak havoc on your skin, leaving it dry, itchy, and flaky. This is certainly something you'd prefer to avoid.

But what is the reason behind these pesky flakes?

And how are you supposed to get rid of them?

More importantly, how do you prevent them from reoccurring?

Inside this book, you will find the answers to all these questions and more. You will also learn how to make your own natural skincare products specifically formulated to combat dry skin.

No longer do you need to worry about dry, flaky skin or what chemicals are being put onto your body.

Each chapter of this book focuses on a different type of skincare product and provides you with multiple recipes. Moreover, every product is part of a skincare routine you can follow for the best results.

Remember to patch test each product before using it on your face so that if you have any adverse reactions you can catch it right away. We'll have so much fun creating these recipes together!

ALL ABOUT DRY SKIN

What Is Dry Skin?

When there isn't enough moisture in the skin, it feels dry. In medical terms, this is known as "xeroderma."

Severely dry skin is called "xerosis."

When you have dry skin, it feels rough and looks scaly. You may also experience itchiness, also known as pruritus, as well as cracks and bleeding in severe cases.

Although dry patches can be caused by a number of conditions, they are generally caused by the lack of moisture in the skin. This is usually solved with a bit of moisturizer. But when these patches are inflamed or irritated, fixing the issue becomes much harder.

Not every dry patch looks the same. Patches of dry skin may feel flaky, crusty, itchy, or scaly, and appear pink or red in color. You can tell where they are by feeling your skin. There will probably be dry patches if there are small raised areas or different textures that feel like rough sandpaper.

What Causes Dry Skin?

Dry, flaky facial skin occurs because of skin dehydration, which has a lot of internal and external causes. There are several factors that contribute to dry facial skin, and the intensity and number of these factors will determine how severe it is.

External Triggers of Dry Skin

Typically, environmental triggers and bad skincare routines ~~that~~ cause dry skin on your face. Generally, dry patches on the face develop due to exposure to these external causes more often than the rest of the body. Let's take a look at what these external factors are.

1. Environmental Factors

- Extreme temperatures: extreme heat, cold, and dryness
- Changing seasons: Winter and summer are the most common times for dry skin symptoms.
- UV Rays: The sun's UV rays can accelerate skin aging, increasing its proneness to dryness as well.
- Chlorine: Dry skin can occur after coming into contact with chlorine in a swimming pool.

2. Skincare

- Skin barrier lipids are stripped away when you wash your face frequently or take long, hot showers.
- The wrong skincare routine can also cause dryness in your skin. The best way to treat dry skin is by adhering to a routine and using products suitable for dry skin, rather than using harsh soaps or serums that may strip the skin of its natural lipids.

3. Medication

Medications may change the balance of water in the skin. This side effect is commonly associated with medications for controlling blood pressure, such as diuretics. If you suspect that a medication is causing dry skin, consult your doctor or pharmacist.

External Factors of Dry Skin: The Causes And Effects

The skin's natural lipid surface barrier deteriorates when it's exposed to all those external factors. The moisture-binding substances in your skin can be washed out once the lipid barrier is broken. If these natural moisture-binding substances are not replenished and the skin's lipid barrier is not repaired, the skin becomes dry as a result and is unable to hold as much water.

In the case of dry skin, if you don't treat it with moisturizing skincare products, your skin's deeper layers can also dry out, which disrupts your moisture networks. Consequently, moisture doesn't flow up into the upper layers, so the skin gets severely dry.

Internal Triggers of Dry Skin

1. The Influence of Genetics

We all have different genes that determine things like what color our skin is, how much moisture it has, and how much lipid it contains. This means that everyone's skin has different moisture and lipid levels, even when subject to the exact same conditions.

People with fair skin tend to have drier skin than people with darker skin due to their genetic composition. Genetics also plays a role in diseases like Psoriasis, Atopic Dermatitis, Ichthyosis, and diabetes.

2. The Influence of Hormones

Our hormones fluctuate during different stages of our lives, such as during adolescence, pregnancy, and menopause. Hence, our skin's moisture balance gets disrupted. Pregnant women often experience dry skin on their faces. Menopause also reduces estrogen levels in the body, resulting in drier skin.

3. UV Radiation

As you get older, your skin ages naturally. Nevertheless, prolonged exposure to ultraviolet rays can speed up the aging process and cause wrinkles and fine lines. In order to prevent premature skin aging, you should avoid overexposure to the sun and protect your skin against UV rays by applying sunscreen daily.

4. Aging

As we get older, our skin produces less sweat and lipids. This is because the sebaceous glands and sweat glands of the skin no longer function as well as they did when we were younger. As the skin ages, it becomes more prone to dryness, leading to wrinkles and fine lines.

Other Factors Causing Dry Skin

In addition to the main causes just mentioned, the severity of facial skin dryness is also affected by several other factors. You can minimize their impact if you are aware of them.

1. Ineffective Treatment

Dry skin is likely to worsen if it is not properly treated or if ineffective moisturizers are used. When the deeper layers of the skin are affected by dryness, their moisture networks are diminished. The upper layers of the skin rely on these networks for moisture, resulting in increased dryness when they are compromised.

2. Risks Associated With the Work or Leisure Activities

Outdoor sports, gardening, and holidays in cold climates, among other activities, can cause dry facial skin. Face dryness caused by environmental and occupational irritants can be dealt with by avoiding these factors, taking appropriate precautions when doing them, and/or using adequate skincare products.

3. Exposure to the Sun

Dry skin on the face can be caused by excessive sun exposure. Choose sunscreen specifically designed for dry skin, and make sure it contains moisturizing ingredients as well as an adequate SPF.

You also need to make sure any product you use on dry skin doesn't contain fragrances or colors that can irritate it. Compared to normal skin, dry skin is more likely to become inflamed and irritated.

4. Dehydration

The amount of moisture in your skin is directly related to the body's ability to supply water. If your body is dehydrated, it can't supply sufficient hydration to the skin, so dry skin develops.

Elderly people, as well as manual workers and athletes, are prone to dehydration due to reducedthirst sensations.

5. Smoking

We all know that smoking is bad for you, but when it comes to your skin, toxins such as nicotine can lower blood flow. Smoking also slows down the metabolism of the skin, resulting in premature aging and dryness. Finally, using tobacco can make your lips irritated.

6. Diet

Our skin needs a variety of different nutrients, vitamins, and unsaturated fatty acids for its proper function. Skin can get dry if you don't get the proper nutrients. Keep your skin healthy by eating a balanced diet.

How to Know if You Have Dry Skin

When you initially start developing dry patches on your skin, it will feel tight and dehydrated. But if you leave it untreated, it will worsen, leading to flaky and even drier skin.

This can turn sore and red. When your skin is dehydrated, it lacks moisture and appears rough and dull.

The T-zone is the area that covers your forehead, nose, chin, and cheeks.

It is more prone to flaky skin and dryness during winter.

When You Have Dry Skin on Your Face

Initially, when your skin starts to lose moisture, you may notice dryness in the form of roughness and/or tightness.

When You Have Extremely Dry Skin on Your Face

When this initial dryness is not treated properly, it progresses and leads to several other conditions, wherein your skin becomes:

- Scaly
- Extremely tight
- Itchy
- Red
- Flaky
- Chapped

There are chances that you might also develop fine lines, which lead to wrinkles and accelerate the aging process. If this gets worse, it can lead to bleeding and peeling. And if you have a darker skin tone, your skin may even look gray and ashy.

When You Have Sensitive Dry Facial Skin

With dry skin comes skin sensitivity. However, that doesn't mean that sensitive skin is always related to dryness. When your skin suffers from both sensitivity and dryness, avoid skincare products that have colorants and fragrances.

When You Have Dry Skin Around Your Eyes

You may have noticed flaky, dry, and itchy skin around your eyes, on your eyelids, and even under your eyes. This is caused by a number of factors such as environmental changes, eczema, and lifestyle choices.

Other Dry Facial Skin Conditions and Diseases

- Psoriasis and Atopic dermatitis are linked to dry skin.
- Hyperthyroidism is another condition that leads to dry, peeling skin. It is a condition in which your thyroid gland doesn't produce enough thyroid hormones.
- Diabetes mellitus and several kidney diseases also lead to dry skin on your face.
- If you have acne and are taking medications, be it topical or oral, you can expect extremely dry skin as a side effect.

Advantages and Disadvantages of Having Dry Skin

If you're feeling discouraged, don't fret. Dry skin isn't all bad!

Dry skin comes with both advantages and disadvantages. Let's take a look at what these are.

Advantages of Dry Skin

1. Attracts Less Dirt

Dry skin doesn't attract as much dirt, dust, and grime when compared to oily skin, since it lacks oil. When dirt settles on oily skin, it tends to block the pores, not allowing them to breathe. This is not the case with dry skin, which makes people with dry skin look fresh for a prolonged time. Therefore, as your skin produces less oil, your skin looks matte and dirt-free.

2. Not Having To Worry About Makeup

People with oily skin often find it difficult to keep their makeup in place. Their makeup will slide off after application since oils don't let makeup sit on the skin for long. But people with dry skin don't face this issue, as a hydrating moisturizer and foundation is enough to keep the makeup in place for a longer time without needing any touch-ups.

3. Fewer Blackheads and Pimples

Blackheads and pimples occur when pores get clogged with dirt and oil, which is why oily skin is more prone to these conditions.

Your dry skin doesn't present those problems, since any moisture you could attract would actually do you good in terms of giving you a healthy glow instead of making you look flaky.

Disadvantages of Dry Skin

1. Difficult to Maintain

Oily skin isn't so difficult to take care of, but with dry skin, there are times when it seems pointless to do anything at all. We sometimes find it stressful to use moisturizer multiple times a day, let alone visit the salon every month.

2. Displays Early Signs of Aging

Wrinkles and aging lines are among the most common problems associated with dry skin. The lack of sebum in your skin causes cracks and lines to appear very quickly, giving your skin wrinkles and lines that are permanent.

If you are over 30, you should begin using anti-aging creams. We shall discuss how to make these anti-aging products later on in the book.

SKINCARE BASICS FOR DRY SKIN

Graceful aging is all about having a good skincare routine.

A baby's skin is smooth, soft, and wrinkle-free. As we age, our skin loses its youthful elasticity and starts to sag. The harsh elements in the environment also cause the skin to become drier and tougher.

A good skincare regimen can be beneficial in slowing down the detrimental effects of time and the environment and improve the health of our skin.

But before you begin with a good skincare routine, you need an understanding of how your skin works.

Three Main Layers of the Skin

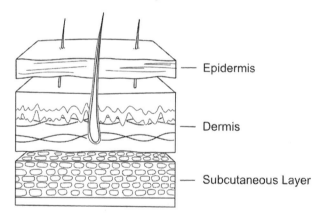

— Epidermis

— Dermis

— Subcutaneous Layer

Our skin consists of three layers. The innermost layer is made of subcutaneous tissue. This tissue consists of fat cells that help to insulate our body. The middle layer of the skin is known as the dermis. This layer consists of connective tissues. And the outermost layer is called the epidermis. This protects our inner skin from environmental elements.

Epidermal cells move continuously from the innermost part of the epidermis to the outermost part of the skin. Once they reach the top, they flake off. As the cells in the epidermis thin out, the skin becomes thinner and loses its elasticity. This leads to your skin getting wrinkled and saggy.

In addition, your sweat glands decrease with age, resulting in drier skin. The aging of your skin also results in smaller cells in the subcutaneous layer, which leads to sagging and wrinkles.

The UVA and UVB radiation that is emitted by sunlight thins the epidermis even further. Additionally, they speed up the collagen breakdown within the dermis.

A good skincare routine must include thorough cleansing and moisturizing. Cleansing your skin is important for getting rid of dead skin cells and dirt. When your skin is clean, it prevents acne from occurring.

Cleansing your skin, however, can also lead to dryness, since it removes the natural oils that help retain hydration. To counteract this, you need a moisturizer. Moisturizing your skin restores the water levels and protects it. It is an essential part of your skincare routine.

For dry skin, you must use a hydrating and moisturizing face cleanser that doesn't strip your skin of its natural oils.

You must also follow it up with a nourishing moisturizer both during the day and the night. If needed, you can also top your moisturizer off with a facial oil.

The Importance of Skincare for Dry Skin

Taking care of your skin is not just for looks. The skin is the largest organ of your body and is important for your overall health.

When you take good care of it, it, in turn, takes good care of you.

Therefore, it is important that you have a well-thought-out skincare routine. Your time, energy, and efforts are absolutely worth it when you take care of your skin on a daily basis.

1. The skin sheds its cells every day.

Yes, your skin sheds its cells EVERY day in order to replenish itself.

It is a natural and necessary process that happens to everyone.

However, the new cells that regenerate need a little help to get the most out of them, which is why even though you do an amazing job on your skincare routine today, you still have to repeat it tomorrow.

2. Your skincare routine will save you money.

Taking care of your skin and its health will help you avoid many issues that can otherwise be extremely costly.

Acne scars, skin discoloration, wrinkles, fine lines, and many other things are all directly related to bad skin health.

A proper skincare routine, when followed regularly, prevents all these issues and consequent trips to a cosmetic surgeon or a dermatologist in the future.

3. Different skin types have different needs.

Different skin types come with their own set of needs and hence require their own skincare routine.

When you have dry skin, you need an added boost of moisturizer and facial oils to combat the dryness.

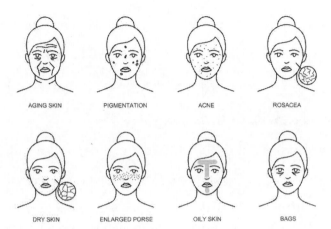

Knowing what type of skincare products suit your skin is very important. Check what your skin needs, what it looks like, and what issues you need to address.

For example, dry skin is more prone to developing dry, itchy, patches and flakes and is often characterized by roughness.

No matter what areas you want to target, this book has the right products for you. We'll learn how to make all-natural skincare products for dry skin in the coming chapters.

But before we get started, make sure you know what your skin is dealing with. And if you don't know, go see a dermatologist right away! You've got nothing to lose by putting yourself first. And your skin would probably thank you if it could talk.

4. It is easier to prevent than it is to correct.

We already know that our skin sheds its cells throughout the day and that the environment can have negative effects on our skin.

When you don't take care of your skin properly, it can cause some serious damage in the future. This damage could be anything from dry skin to deep wrinkles to acne scars.

The good news is, you can prevent these and many other skin problems with a proper skincare routine.

It may seem tedious to use cleansers, serums, and moisturizers twice a day, but think about it this way. Would you rather spend 5-10 minutes twice a day, or need to buy expensive treatments in the future?

5. Taking time for yourself is important.

Skincare is not just limited to applying products to your face. It goes hand in hand with self-care.

In this day and age, it is crucial for us to take care of ourselves in regard to our physical, spiritual, mental, and emotional health.

You can use your skincare routine to take some time for yourself and reflect.

Get away from your screens and practice mindfulness while you take care of yourself.

6. You will gain more self-confidence.

Today, not many people are comfortable in their own skin. They often relate their looks and how they present themselves with their confidence.

A person with dry patches, discoloration, and other skin issues might not feel confident enough to step out with their natural skin. They might look for ways to conceal their flaws in order to "feel confident."

Not that makeup is the bad guy, but associating our appearance with how we feel is common, so if you constantly feel the need to cover up your natural skin, you may be harming your self-confidence.

Having clean and clear skin keeps you looking your best naturally, which is definitely a confidence booster.

When you meet someone, one of the first things they notice is your face, so it makes sense for you to put your best face forward.

Following a good skincare routine helps you achieve exactly this!

7. *Taking care of your skin contributes to a healthy lifestyle.*

Taking the time to look after your skin contributes to building daily healthy habits, and these things have a way of snowballing.

Those that start the day with a natural skincare routine are likely to make other healthier choices throughout the rest of their day when it comes to things like hair care, oral care, nutrition, and exercise.

All these combined automatically lead to a better lifestyle, and a happier, and healthier you!

8. *You will have younger-looking skin.*

As we age, the cell turnover of our skin slows down, which makes our skin look dull and less radiant.

When you use high-quality, natural products and follow a skincare routine daily, it helps to get rid of dead skin cells.

This way, your body replaces them with newer cells that are more youthful.

8. You will have younger-looking skin.

As we age, the cell turnover of our skin slows down, which makes our skin look dull and less radiant.

When you use high-quality, natural products and follow a skincare routine daily, it helps to get rid of dead skin cells.

This way, your body replaces them with newer cells that are more youthful.

Debunking Common Myths Around Dry Skin

Dry skin always means you're dehydrated, right?

Wrong!

And you can get rid of the dryness if you drink loads of water, right?

Wrong again!

These are just a couple of myths when it comes to dry skin, but there are many more.

In this section, we will bust some of the most common myths about dry skin so that you can learn how to properly take care of dry skin.

1. When your skin is dry, it's dehydrated.

Dry skin and dehydrated skin are two different skin concerns, though they can be linked to one another.

Dehydrated skin is a result of a lack of non-moisturizing factors (NMF) and hyaluronic acid in your skin. All skin types can be dehydrated—even oily skin.

Dry skin, in contrast, lacks natural lipids in its outer layer, which is known as the stratum corneum. If you want your dry skin to stay moisturized and feel soft and smooth, it needs a healthy balance of lipids. A lack of lipids causes the skin to lose its ability to lock in moisture, resulting in dry skin that is scaly, flaky, red, itchy, and irritated.

To know if your skin is dehydrated, you can perform a pinch test.

1. Pinch your cheek gently and hold it for a moment.
2. If you notice your skin snapping quickly, it is not dehydrated.
3. If your skin takes some time to bounce back, it is dehydrated.

2. You can get rid of dry skin if you drink more water.

This myth is so common that people actually drink liters and liters of water to compensate for the dryness!

Of course, if you drink eight glasses of water every day it helps keep your skin healthy, and provides many other health benefits, but it is most effective on dehydrated skin, not on dry skin that lacks moisture due to an inadequate protective barrier.

3. You get dry skin only during cold weather.

It's true that your skin gets drier when the air is cold, dry, and lacking humidity, but cold air alone is not responsible for your dry skin. Even during summer, intense UV rays, air conditioners, chlorine, and saltwater take a toll on the health of your skin. If you have warmer air with lower humidity, it can contribute to dry and flaky skin as well. You can keep the environment indoors moist during the colder months by using a humidifier. It will not only humidify your skin, but it will also keep it healthy.

4. Moisturizers with a thicker consistency are more hydrating.

It's not about the thickness, it is all about the ingredients.

You might think your dry skin craves a heavier, thicker moisturizer, but the truth is that moisturizers with a gel-based formula are better at hydrating your skin. The gel-like consistency allows the moisturizer to penetrate into the skin faster, keeping your skin hydrated for a longer time.

You want your moisturizer to work deep down in the skin layers. Look for ingredients such as shea butter, squalane, reishi mushroom, and hyaluronic acid in your moisturizer. These ingredients mimic the natural oils present in your skin and increase hydration without clogging your pores.

5. You shouldn't exfoliate dry skin.

Every skin type needs to be exfoliated regularly. When your skin is flaky and dry, serums and moisturizers will not penetrate into your skin and therefore cannot provide the needed hydration. Using a gentle exfoliator at least once a week ensures that the dead skin cells are buffed away so that your skin can soak up all the beneficial ingredients from your skincare products.

Exfoliation also helps get rid of the impurities in your pores. Instead of skipping exfoliation altogether, use an exfoliating cleanser or a cream to get rid of these pesky impurities. Once you are done buffing that top layer, the skincare products you use afterward will be easily absorbed and provide your skin with maximum benefits.

6. Feeding your skin with more oils does the trick.

Dry skin might occur from a lack of natural oils on your skin, but it also needs to be moisturized well. Your skin needs a balance of both nourishment and hydration, which is why you should use a moisturizer during the day and a facial oil at night.

7. Dry skin benefits from hot showers.

A good hot shower at the end of the day may feel relaxing and comforting, but this can come at the expense of skin damage.

Your blood vessels dilate under hot showers, which strips natural oils from your skin. This leads to drier skin. Instead, take showers with lukewarm water and limit your shower time.

8. You can prevent dry skin by layering moisturizers.

No matter how many moisturizers or oils you apply on your skin at once, if they don't contain the right ingredients or aren't able to penetrate your skin effectively, they won't work.

Moisturizers need to have the right ingredients to be effective on dry skin. Use products that are hypoallergenic and chemical-free, since some chemicals can lead to even more irritated skin.

9. Soaps help keep your skin moist and soft.

While soap can temporarily make your skin feel bouncy and soft, they actually strip your skin of moisture. This, in turn, leads to dry skin. Hence, try to avoid soaps on your face, and if you are using one, make sure that it has nourishing ingredients and is tailor-made for dry skin.

SKINCARE ROUTINE FOR DRY SKIN

Now that we have discussed the importance of a skincare routine for dry skin and debunked some myths around it, let's learn more about the steps that go into this specific routine and how you can develop the perfect one according to your needs.

Every skincare routine and each step inside it is unique and important. Skincare, in recent times, has become so popular on social media that we often get confused as to what's trending and what isn't, not to mention what works and what doesn't. On top of that, thousands of new products are launched every year, which makes it even more confusing to get started.

Understanding what ingredients to choose, what kind of products work best for your skin, and how to create a personalized skincare routine is understandably overwhelming.

But that's where this book comes in!

In this chapter, you will learn the different steps in a skincare routine, how to layer products correctly, and how to make your routine effective for your dry skin.

If you're a beginner, this section helps you get started from scratch.

And if you've already indulged in one routine and wish to learn about adding those extra steps or learn how to layer products correctly to make your skincare more effective, we've got you covered too!

Skincare—What It's All About

As the word suggests, "skincare" refers to taking care of your skin.

Our skin protects us from external environmental factors and pathogens that cause damage to our internal organs, so it is extremely important that we protect it and keep it clean and healthy.

Just as you regularly brush your teeth, you must give regular attention to your skin to keep it functioning well.

Proper skin care will also help prevent skin cancer and other skin diseases. When we discuss skincare in this book, know that it refers not only to improving your skin's appearance, but also its functionality.

Skincare—Why Care?

It is important that you give your skin some love for medical as well as cosmetic benefits.

You can't stop how fast time passes by, but by following a proper skincare routine, you can prevent different signs of aging including sun damage, fine lines, wrinkles, and dark spots. You can also prevent other minor skin concerns like excessive dryness or oiliness.

If you've been dealing with rosacea, eczema, psoriasis, or dry patches, skincare is definitely not optional, and you'll want to think about the ingredients that go into your products to ensure that they provide the right level of protection.

But what if you have multiple skin issues?

To target one skin issue, you may need to follow a certain routine with targeted products, but the ingredients in them may make your skin sensitive to other conditions.

So what do you do to target several skin conditions at once?

You follow a balanced skincare routine that targets multiple skin conditions that not only treats but also prevents the symptoms from reoccurring.

And as we have already discussed, taking care of your skin offers mental health benefits. It can also motivate you to live a healthier lifestyle in general.

However, you must remember a few things before you get started with your skincare routine.

Things to Keep In Mind Before Starting a New Skin Care Regimen

We're often excited to try out something new, especially when it comes to skincare and makeup. After all… it's fun! From testing out the product to sniffing the fragrance, it's a beautiful feeling!

But the downside of trying out something new is that you may not get the results you desire.

Changing your skincare routine can be daunting, especially when you are a beginner.

To make things easier, I've compiled some tips to keep in mind before you get started on your new skincare journey.

1. A normal skin reaction and an allergic reaction are different.

Your skin is bound to react, irrespective of whether your skin is happy with the new formulation you have made or not. This reaction can be in the form of mild burning, itching, stinging, or swelling. These reactions are normal and can be expected from using certain ingredients, such as those present in an acidic toner.

On the other hand, an allergic reaction is long-lived and can even be painful. They are not just mere side effects of using a product. If you are in doubt, stop using that product immediately and contact your dermatologist.

If a face wash (or any product, for that matter), stings your eyes, wash it off immediately.

2. Give your skin some time to get adjusted to your skincare routine.

When you start out with your new skincare routine or any new product, observe how your skin talks back to you. Check if there are any reactions, flakiness, dry skin, or acne. If you notice your skin getting dry, irritated, or red, this may have simply resulted from applying serums or moisturizers. In this case, you can reduce the frequency of usage of that specific product. For example, use it only one to three times a week. Give your skin some break between applications and let it get adjusted to the products.

3. Using active ingredients in your skincare takes a minimum of two months to show results.

Imagine you have a first date that doesn't go so well, but you enjoyed texting the following day, so you agree to meet for drinks again. A similar mentality applies to new skincare products you try. You need to give them another chance to see if your skin is compatible with the product or not.

Skincare products such as serums, moisturizers, and skin treatments that contain active ingredients take at least two months to show results.

4. Tingling is not always an indication that the product is working.

Beauty doesn't come with pain, but a little tingling sensation with some products can mean that it is working well on your skin. And this is a happy indicator. You may have noticed that some beauty products, such as face masks or topical creams, often come with a warning label on them about skin tingling being a side effect.

But a tingling sensation is a sign that it is working only when that is the goal of that specific product. Chemical skin peels and acids, for example, can sting and tingle on your skin, resulting in immediate inflammation of the skin. This results in your skin peeling, which is what is meant to happen.

Retinoids also work in a similar fashion. They cause inflammation to your skin and exfoliate it. This encourages the growth of new cells and collagen.

Keep in mind that there is a fine balance between the two. Skincare products should generally not cause any stinging and irritation. When they do, they accelerate skin aging by breaking down the collagen in your skin.

5. Learn when to stop using a product.

Pay attention to which parts of your face you will be treating with your new skincare regimen. If any of the points around your eyes or cheeks feel weird or uncomfortable, consult your dermatologist as soon as possible.

Stop using anything that gives you an allergic reaction, such as swelling of your eyelids, lips, or hives. Avoid using a product that makes you more sensitive to the sun at times when you may be more likely to burn, such as during your summer vacation.

If you experience burning, redness, or swelling with any product you use, stop using it. Consult your dermatologist to determine if any of the ingredients are allergenic. If yu stll have an adverse reaction several days after discontinuing use of the product, contact your dermatologist again.

6. Follow an ideal skincare routine.

Skincare isn't complicated. There is an ideal routine that you should follow so that the products you use get absorbed by your skin and work in the most effective manner. The three basic steps included in the routine are cleansing, moisturizing, and sunscreen. For sunscreen, make sure to use a minimum of SPF 30 and look for a "broad spectrum" label.

This is your morning skincare routine, and you shouldn't skip it. You can also use a moisturizer that has SPF 30 in it to combine the two steps together.

Whatever sunscreen you use, make sure that you use it consistently every single day. It might take you some trial and error to determine the one that suits you, since not every sunscreen you use will blend with your makeup and/or skin tone.

On the other hand, your nighttime skincare routine can include additional steps. If you wear makeup during the day, a cleanser may not be sufficient to remove the makeup and sunscreen from your face. It might even leave your skin feeling sticky and greasy.

In this case, you need to double-cleanse your skin. Start by using an oil-based cleanser to break down the makeup and sunscreen. Follow it up with your regular cleanser to remove the rest of the impurities. You can also use a cotton pad soaked in micellar water before you use a cleanser to get rid of any makeup residue. Double cleansing is recommended when you have sunscreen and/or makeup on during the day, but it isn't a necessity otherwise.

Once you cleanse your skin, follow it up with a toner, serum, and moisturizer. You could use your daytime moisturizer at night, but since you don't have to worry about applying makeup or sunscreen at night, a thicker moisturizer may be better suited for this step.

In the specific case of dry skin, use a hydrating moisturizer and top it off with facial oil at night.

Building the Perfect Skincare Routine

Building the perfect skincare routine can be tricky for a beginner. Getting into skincare can often be like going down a rabbit hole, especially in these times, when so many of us are looking for new ways to keep ourselves busy. However, adding more and more steps and products to your routine can be overwhelming and stressful, which is the exact opposite of what your grooming routine should do for you. So before you take any of this skincare advice, try to be realistic about what you can commit to.

Take these tips seriously, and you will age with grace for the rest of your life. But more important than that is the sense of satisfaction that comes with taking care of yourself on a daily basis.

This chapter will help you to design a personalized skincare routine that will take you no more than five to ten minutes each morning and evening. And if multiple steps are too much, you can even just start with a simple CTM (cleanser, toner, moisturizer) routine, and see how it goes.

If you have dry skin, you will achieve the best results if you develop and stick to a new skincare regimen that moisturizes your skin and keeps it hydrated.

This skincare routine is divided into three parts: morning, evening, and weekly.

The morning skincare routine ensures that your skin is not damaged by the sun and pollutants during the day, while the evening routine helps reverse any damage caused by the sun and pollution during the day. The weekly skincare routine gives your skin some TLC by exfoliating the dead skin cells, pollution, and dirt, as well as rejuvenating your skin.

But before we discuss these skincare routines, let us first understand how to layer the products correctly.

How to Correctly Layer Skincare Products

Typically, you will find that a basic skincare routine consists of cleansing, moisturizing, and sunscreen—but what if you have additional steps in your routine? Obviously, you need to layer serums, toners, creams, and moisturizers in some order, but there is so much conflicting information that it is difficult to decide which products you need and in what order to use them.

It's generally recommended to order products based on texture and pH level—lighter products should be applied before creams with heavier textures, and lower pH products should be applied before higher pH products. Various products are absorbed in different ways, and as a result, their efficacy can be determined by the order in which they are applied.

Yet, to what extent can these rules actually be applied to real life?

When layering your products, keep the following things in mind.

Consistency Matters

We all know that oil and water don't mix well.

A product's water content has a greater impact on its absorption than anything else. A water-based product can usually be layered on top of another without affecting the penetration of either.

You can't layer water-based products on top of oil-based products (such as ointments, creams, or serums) because water won't penetrate them.

In other words, use water-based products first, followed by oil-based products.

pH Matters

For cosmetic purposes, pH—or how acidic the skincare product is—also matters.

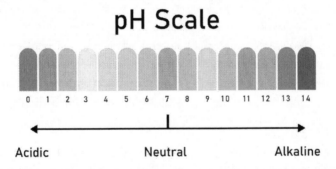

The majority of active ingredients, except benzoyl peroxide, have acidic pH values below 5. Also, the pH of your skin is naturally slightly below 5 (just below neutral), which has a direct impact on the pH of anything it comes in contact with.

When you apply a pH 4 serum over a pH 3 one, which is again applied over a pH 4.5 serum, it creates a mix of different pH levels, and not just in the middle of 3 and 4.

So, How Do You Layer Products?

When you apply multiple products to your skin, it doesn't mean they form layers on your skin when absorbed. They all get absorbed at the same time. But if you give one product some time—about a minute or two—before you apply the next one, you can allow your skin to completely absorb each product.

Morning Skincare Routine for Dry Skin

Following a morning skincare routine ensures that your skin is protected from harmful UV rays and contaminants.

Here is a skincare routine that you can follow on a day-to-day basis to help your dry skin.

1. Cleanser

Begin your morning skincare routine with a gentle, yet effective cleanser that helps clear away dirt and other impurities from your skin without drying it out.

For dry skin, an ideal cleanser is one that has an oil-based or cream-based formula. This will ensure that your skin stays hydrated and soft. You can use one that has glycerin and other nourishing ingredients to moisturize your skin. We'll learn how to make cleansers in the coming chapters.

2. Toner

Once you cleanse your skin, you need a toner to balance your skin. It helps prep your skin for all other ingredients

After cleansing your face, choose a well-formulated toner to balance your skin.

A toner helps prepare your skin for the next steps in your skincare routine, so it is an essential step after washing your face. Dry skin needs toner that not only hydrates but also restores skin, balances pH levels, and exfoliates. Hyaluronic acid, glycerin, and aloe vera are some of the ingredients you can include in your toner to lock in hydration and moisture.

3. Serum

A damaged moisture barrier can cause your skin to dry out, so if you have dry skin, you probably have a damaged barrier. Use a serum that contains niacinamide, ceramides, and probiotics to protect and rebuild your skin barrier.

Your skincare routine shouldn't be complete without serums, which you'll want to apply after toner. Choose a serum that provides moisture to dry skin and shields it from environmental aggressors like pollution.

Here are a few ingredients that you can consider in your serums:

- Hyaluronic acid: Hyaluronic acid helps the skin retain moisture.
- Ceramides: Ceramides form a moisture-retaining barrier on the skin.
- Squalane: Squalane is a naturally occurring lipid found in the skin that helps to retain moisture.
- Vitamin C: As an antioxidant, vitamin C stimulates collagen production, wards off environmental aggressors, and thickens the dermis.
- Plant oils and extracts: Shea butter, coconut oil, and jojoba oil help seal in moisture to the skin.

4. Moisturizer

Everyone's skincare routine should include moisturizing, regardless of the time of day.

To maintain soft and hydrated skin all day long, make sure your moisturizer has hydrating ingredients, like ceramides and hyaluronic acid.

Remember that cold weather can affect your skin, which is why you might want to use a moisturizer with a thicker consistency during the winter months.

Dry skin requires a moisturizer that contains rich, nourishing ingredients that penetrate deeply into the skin's barrier. This will make your skin more supple, smooth, and plump.

The ingredients in a good face moisturizer for dry skin may also include hyaluronic acid, ceramides, glycerin, and B vitamins like niacinamide. These ingredients can fade spots, reduce redness, and restore evenness to your skin, regardless of whether you suffer from acne or wrinkles.

5. Eye Cream

You must also remember to apply eye cream if you have dry skin. You should apply a small amount from under the eyes and below the brows, over your eyelids. Take extra care of the skin around your eyes, since it is particularly sensitive.

With the right eye cream, you can prevent problems such as fatigue, dryness, and other signs of aging. Your skincare routine should include a lightweight eye cream with nourishing ingredients. Moisture can be retained and restored with ingredients such as vitamin B, collagen, vitamin C, shea butter, and hyaluronic acid.

6. Sunscreen

Sunscreen is an essential part of any skincare routine. You should apply it every day during the day after your moisturizer. Wearing sunscreen is especially important when you have dry skin, as harsh UV rays can leave your skin stressed, dehydrated, and unbalanced. If you're going to spend a lot of time outdoors in the sun, reapply it often, about once every 2-3 hours.

Consider using a lightweight sunscreen that doesn't cause breakouts or clog pores. Sadly, even dry skin can experience this. Make sure the sunscreen you use has an SPF of at least 30.

7. Lip Balm

The last step of your morning skincare routine is using a lip balm. Our lips do not have sebaceous glands, and hence, it is important to moisturize them as well. Not moisturizing them will result in dry, chapped, and flaky lips, which may even bleed.

A lip balm will keep your lips moisturized, soft, and hydrated for a long time. You can even reapply them every few hours to ensure that moisture isn't lost.

If you are stepping out and wish to skip lipstick, you can use a tinted lip balm. This will add a hint of color to your lips while still moisturizing them.

Evening Skin Care Routine for Dry Skin

Our skin repairs and rejuvenates itself while we sleep, and hence, the skincare routine we follow at night plays a crucial role in the appearance and health of our skin.

1. Cleanser

Cleansers are a must to remove your makeup at the end of the day. But you should also cleanse your face, even if you don't have makeup on. Using a cleanser before going to bed makes sure that your skin is free from excess oil, dirt, and impurities. Clean skin ensures that your skin can absorb the nutrients from the products in the following steps of your routine.

Cleansing balms or oils are better for dry skin than gels and foam formulas to melt away makeup, impurities, and sunscreen effectively. These will not dry out your skin and strip off the moisture.

2. Toner

Applying toner is as important at night as it is in the morning. It not only removes any leftover makeup, impurities, or sunscreen but is also the first step of hydration that provides your skin with an added boost of moisture before you layer it on with a serum and moisturizer. Make sure that you include nourishing ingredients instead of acid-based formulas, since the latter can greatly dry out your skin.

3. Targeted Treatments Like Serums, Ampoules, and Essences

You can use the same serum you used for your daytime routine for your nighttime routine. However, if you want to target specific concerns, use a concentrated serum or a treatment.

If your skin is dry and/or dehydrated, layer on a hyaluronic acid serum underneath your moisturizer. Hyaluronic acid attracts moisture to the skin and prevents it from evaporating. Additionally, the molecules hold 1,000 times their weight in water, maximizing the hydrating effect of your other products.

4. Moisturizer

It's okay to use a heavier moisturizer at night, since your face won't get shiny, and it won't feel heavy. Make sure you apply a thicker, richer night cream if your day cream is thinner. Use creamy, thick formulas with ingredients like ceramides, peptides, and oat lipids instead of gel-based formulas.

5. Eye Cream

Your dry skin skincare routine should include an eye cream specially formulated for the sensitive skin around your eyes. Using this can help treat issues such as puffy eyes and dark circles. If you want to limit dark circles and fine lines around the eyes, use an eye cream that has anti-aging properties. If you want to reduce hyperpigmentation around your eyes, you should use a vitamin C-enriched eye cream.

6. Facial Oil

This step seals in all the moisturizing ingredients you just applied. It has been recommended by dermatologists and estheticians as a method of treating dry skin, especially during the winter. Spend time massaging a face oil or balm into the skin in order to increase absorption and blood circulation. If you prefer, you can use a gua sha to apply it and massage your face.

Applying facial oil adds that extra layer of moisture, which is crucial for dry skin. If you prefer, you can also use it during the day. However, make sure that you use one with a lighter consistency during the day and a heavier one during the night.

You can use an oil that has antioxidant ingredients such as vitamin C and vitamin E.

7. Lip Balm

Do not sleep without applying lip balm! You can use a thicker lip balm before going to bed to wake up with soft, smooth, and hydrated lips.

8. Bonus Step: Overnight Mask

Instead of facial oil, you can also use a nourishing leave-on mask as the last step in your skincare regimen. This will seal in all the powerful nutrients that you've applied throughout your routine.

As you sleep, overnight masks replenish the cells in your skin and hydrate it, boosting moisture levels.

Apply this mask as the last step, once you are done using all other products. When you wake up, wash off the mask before you apply any other product.

Various overnight masks are beneficial for dry skin. If you want your skin to be smoother and softer over time, use one with hyaluronic acid or antioxidants.

Weekly Routine for Dry Skin

1. Exfoliation

The idea of exfoliating dry skin might seem counterintuitive, right? It seems like exfoliating a parched complexion will just make it worse. But that's not the case!

When we busted the myth about exfoliating dry skin, we learned how important it is to exfoliate dry skin.

Keeping dry skin healthy and hydrated requires exfoliating the dead skin flakes.

However, you should choose a gentle exfoliator, one that has spherical, evenly-shaped beads and not pointed ones. This will prevent any damage and microtears on your skin. You can also use one that has AHAs to further benefit your dry skin.

Glycolic acid is one such AHA that encourages healthy skin turnover by removing dead cells from the top layer of the skin.

Make sure you follow up with a moisturizer and SPF, since glycolic acid makes your skin more prone to sun damage.

2. Face Mask

Face masks, especially those formulated for dry skin, provide focused, potent, and much-needed moisturization to combat dryness. Using hydrating and deep-penetrating masks are incredible for dry skin that has a rough, uneven texture, and is flaky, peeling, and cracked. These masks also help to minimize the appearance of fine lines, wrinkles, and other signs of aging.

Do not apply masks with harsh ingredients on your dry skin. Make sure that your mask has a humectant, an ingredient that holds onto water, as this will best hydrate your skin.

WHY HOMEMADE NATURAL SKINCARE IS BETTER

As more and more people are becoming aware that putting ingredients they cannot pronounce on their faces may be harmful over time, they are rethinking the products they buy and use.

Let's take a look at some harmful ingredients that are in conventional skincare products.

Harmful Ingredients in Skincare Products

The skin has a protective barrier that prevents harsh elements from affecting it, which means the body does not necessarily absorb all products applied to the skin. Only a very small proportion of products are actually absorbed by the skin in the form of small molecules. Water molecules, for instance, do not absorb well, and many other molecules in skincare products are either not absorbed at all, or very slowly.

Often, the synthetic ingredients found in these products act as "vehicles" to make sure the active ingredients get absorbed deep into the skin. Without this, some ingredients wouldn't get absorbed by the skin, making the product ineffective.

So, are these synthetic materials harmful?

Well, yes, possibly.

There are many potentially harmful ingredients in commercial skincare products, including preservatives and pesticides, chemicals, parabens, sulfates, and more...

The aim of natural skincare is to move away from these harmful ingredients and avoid using them on our skin.

Now, there is a problem that arises with the natural skincare products available on the market. The ingredients found in products branded as "natural" are not regulated, which means they may contain the same potentially harmful synthetic ingredients as those that are present in other similar products.

For the average consumer, it becomes challenging to know what to buy since there are so many products with different ingredients on the market. How are we to know what is harmful and what isn't?

Even when we find a product that claims to be 100% organic and all-natural, it most likely won't come with a guarantee that it won't lead to skin irritation. That's where this book comes in.

Why People Are Shifting Towards Natural Skincare

Consumers are stepping away from traditional skincare products in favor of their natural alternatives. We want to avoid synthetic chemicals that may be harmful. Natural ones promise better, gentler results for people who have had bad experiences with commercially available products.

Natural solutions also appeal to customers who wish to reflect their values in their purchasing habits. Alternatively, they may see natural products as a way to reconnect with nature, or even as a way to return to something a little simpler and more dependable—perhaps they are simply looking for cleaner, thoughtful products. Using natural products provides a connection to our deeper values in a world where we feel disconnected, hurried, and out of touch. Increasingly, people are choosing natural solutions that help them build a sense of connection to nature, responsibility, and awareness. It's simple: We want our actions and purchases to reflect who we are and who we want to be.

These days, information about where our consumable products are made is much easier to access thanks to computers, the internet, and social media. You can look up all the nasty chemicals present in beauty products (such as parabens, SLS, SLES, and PEGs) online. All the information is at your fingertips.

The need for animal-based ingredients and petroleum-based ingredients is being questioned: Why would I use a petroleum-based product on my skin? Is it necessary to use something synthetic and potentially toxic? Is there another option that would do less or no damage and still give me the best outcome?

When people look at the ingredients list of a product marketed as natural, they are often surprised to learn that they still contain a whole bunch of not-so-nice things. Even though these things are labeled as natural, you may still have questions: What exactly is "natural?" What does it even mean? If nature can already provide us with the necessary building blocks for our existence, why do we need synthetic ingredients?

So, what is your take on natural skincare?

If you wish to reduce your carbon footprint and switch to a cleaner, more natural skincare routine, give it a shot! However, don't feel pressured to throw all your synthetic products immediately in the trash. What is important is that you find out what works best for your skin.

But how effective is homemade skincare?

Well, it all depends on how you formulate the products, what ingredients you use, and how you use them.

Many cultures around the world have a long tradition of creating homemade skincare products, with recipes that are often handed down from generation to generation. The green beauty movement has led to a revival of homemade skincare in recent years. DIY-ing homemade skincare has become a booming trend.

However, there are a few things you must consider before you start making skincare products at home. It's important to maximize the use of your natural ingredients so that they don't go to waste and, more importantly, that your products are safe to use.

Things to Keep In Mind Before Making Skincare Products at Home

1. Select the Right Homemade Skincare Formulation

Creating homemade skincare products begins with finding an effective formula—one that nourishes the skin and also remains stable once it has been applied. The formulation you select should take into account not just the components, but also how those components interact with each other once combined. Ingredients are what make up the formulation. Of course, you want to use only the best botanical ingredients when making your own skincare products. It's exciting to choose from a wide range of smooth and creamy exotic butters, mineral-rich clays, the heady aromas of the essential oils, a wide range of cold-pressed plant oils, the gentle and soothing flower waters, and the list goes on and on...

It will be necessary for you to find a professional formulation after you have decided on the ingredients you wish to use. As there is a lot of information out there that contains dangerous beauty recipes, it can be difficult to find safe and reputable recipes for homemade skincare.

Lastly, it is important to keep in mind that not all formulations can be created at home. Some products require both cosmetic science and technical expertise in order to be made safely and in accordance with various regulations and guidelines, so it's best to buy those from a trusted retailer.

2. Include a Natural Preservative System

Cosmetic products are usually enriched with preservatives so that they can last longer. Most of the products containing water—and even the ones that are anhydrous, meaning that they don't contain water or hydrophilic (water-loving) ingredients—need a preservative system to protect them from bacteria, molds, and yeast.

Your preservative system must be a broad spectrum in nature, which means it should protect your formulation from the growth of bacteria—both gram-positive and gram-negative bacteria, molds, and yeast.

You can easily find natural preservatives, and we'll take a look at them as we formulate the products.

But that's not all!

You also need microbiology and stability tests to determine the expiration date of your skincare products. These tests also ascertain if the preservative system you used works as it should.

All this testing for homemade products sounds like a difficult step, but there are several very simple tests that you can do to ensure the safety of your formulation.

Be extremely careful with formulations that contain water, honey, clay, and fruits. These ingredients are likely to spoil quicker than others and need a suitable, strong, and natural preservative system. This ensures that the product remains stable and safe for its desired shelf life.

Organic skin care formulators often choose to create homemade skin care products that are waterless to limit the growth of microbes, which is why they typically choose to use anhydrous products. However, remember that anhydrous formulations are often prone to rancidity and oxidation. To slow down these processes of degradation, you need to add an antioxidant in your formulation, like vitamin E.

Also, keep in mind that contamination can also occur even before you can visibly notice any signs of microbial or fungal growth in your product. Therefore, if you do not wish to add preservatives to your formula, even natural ones, you must stick to creating only anhydrous products.

In a nutshell, you just need to keep two things in mind:

1. Use an antioxidant for anhydrous products, since they are prone to oxidation.

2. Use a preservative system for water-containing products, since they are prone to contamination.

3. Select the Right Kind of Container

Selecting gorgeous packaging for your homemade skincare products is, of course, exciting and fun! The right kind of packaging will also ensure that your formulation remains stable and safe for a longer time. It is crucial to store your skincare products in hygienic, properly-sealed containers. There are many suppliers that have ready-to-use containers that you can choose to use for your formulations.

Even if the container does have a proper seal, when you have to open it completely, it increases the risk of contamination. Consider using nozzles or spray valves that will disperse your formula from the bottle without requiring you to open the container.

The viscosity of the product may make it impractical to use a pump or spray, so if that is the case, you can consider adding either a spatula or a drop dispenser to reduce the chance of contamination.

4. Make the Right Amount of Product

It is extremely difficult to predict the expiry date of homemade skincare products, so it is recommended to only create small amounts at a time. You'll not only get to use the freshest creams, balms, or butter by doing this, but you'll also be able to experiment with new ingredients more frequently.

With anhydrous products, you can produce larger quantities as long as they are packaged properly to minimize contaminants. Make sure you add antioxidants like rosemary, CO_2, or vitamin E extract to delay degradation.

In the right conditions, microbes can grow very quickly, so you should only make single-use quantaties of unpreserved, water-based products as and when they are required.

5. Make Sure to Properly Measure Ingredients

Exact measurements of your ingredients in appropriate quantities are crucial while making skincare products. Measure both solids and liquids by weight using a high-quality weighing scale/machine.

One more thing to keep in mind is that the volume of your liquid ingredients tends to vary depending on their temperature and density. You can easily exceed the concentration recommended if you measure them in drops. This can happen especially while using essential oils that need to be added in low concentrations.

It is also a good idea to write down your formula and use percentages. This way you can either scale it to a bigger amount or reproduce your batch.

6. Follow the Recommendations for Usage

One of the primary reasons people decide to make their own skincare products is so that they know exactly what they're putting on their skin. Not only are the ingredients used in the formula important, but also how one uses the product. It is important to follow the correct usage recommendations.

When you make your skincare products, certain ingredients, such as carrier oils, can be used in their 100% concentration. On the other hand, there are ingredients that come with strict dose recommendations.

Remember that when you work with essential oils, you need to consider dermal limits. The same is true when using preservatives. You must follow the usage level recommended for effectiveness and safety.

Natural preservatives and essential oils are the ingredients that lead to sensitization in people. Hence, it is crucial that you follow the recommended usage limits by the manufacturer or supplier to make sure that your products safe.

7. Measure the pH

Another important step that you must not miss while making skin-care products is measuring the pH of your product. This is crucial for your product's safety.

Several important properties of your formulation will be influenced by the pH of your product. The pH indicates, for example, whether a particular preservative is effective and safe. A product's pH also affects, among other attributes, its appearance, feel, colors and scents.

To measure the pH of your homemade skincare products, there is no need for a high-tech pH meter; pH strips are an easy and inexpensive way to start formulating and testing your own skincare products.

8. Have Good Manufacturing Practices (GMP)

When making homemade skincare products, a major concern is being sure not to contaminate the product during any stage of production and usage.

A Good Manufacturing Practice, or GMP, calls for routinely cleaning and disinfecting your equipment, containers, and working areas, washing your hands, and using protective gear, such as lab gloves, to protect yourself.

NATURAL CLEANSER RECIPES

1. Aloe Vera and Rosehip Nourishing Cleanser

Aloe vera is well known as an effective antibacterial, anti-inflammatory, and wound healing agent. It is typically used to treat sunburns and other skin concerns because it contains an abundance of enzymes, antioxidants, and vitamins A, C, and E.

This face cleanser contains aloe vera to help soothe your skin, keep inflammation at bay, and balance the microbiome on your skin—all of which leads to radiant, glowing skin.

Ingredients Needed:

- ½ cup aloe vera gel (for fresh aloe vera gel, take aloe and make a purée in a food processor before you start making the cleanser)
- ½ cup rose water (you can add more or less rose water depending on what consistency you prefer)
- 2 tablespoons Castile soap
- 4 drops of rosehip essential oil
- 4 drops of lavender essential oil
- 2 teaspoons argan oil
- 8-ounce squeeze bottle or pump bottle

Instructions:

1. Mix all ingredients together and pour into the bottle using a funnel.
2. Combine the ingredients by tightly screwing on the lid and shaking well.
3. Your cleanser is ready to use!

Notes:

- If using fresh aloe vera gel, refrigerate it and use it within a week.
- In the case of store-bought aloe vera, it should last for one month without refrigeration.
- Any time you notice a change in smell or texture, replace it with a new batch.

How to Use the Cleanser:

1. Shake the cleanser well before use, as the ingredients may separate.
2. Wet your face and take a pea-sized amount on your hands.
3. Rub it to create a lather and gently massage it onto your skin. Make sure to avoid your eyes and lips.
4. Rinse your face off with cool water.

Benefits of Ingredients Used:

1. Aloe Vera Gel

- Reduces acne and blemishes

Aloe vera is effective for fighting acne by acting as an antibacterial and anti-inflammatory agent. It stops pimples and acne from forming by preventing bacteria build-up, as well as speeding up the healing process. Additionally, it eliminates all the blemishes and scars left by acne.

- Hydrates and soothes dry, flaky skin

Aloe vera is renowned as a natural moisturizer. The gel hydrates the skin and gets absorbed quickly. Due to its light texture, aloe vera works well even on oily and acne-prone skin.

- Relieves skin irritation

The cooling properties in aloe vera gel help soothe sunburn, irritated skin, rashes, infections, and redness. It is therefore excellent for sensitive skin. Additionally, its antifungal properties can be used to treat summer heat boils and cysts.

- Reduces the signs of aging

Often, aging signs become more noticeable on the face as elasticity is lost in the skin. Some examples include smile lines, crow's feet, and sagging necks. Aloe vera gel keeps your skin moisturized and restores its radiance. It improves the elasticity of the skin and repairs damaged skin cells. This not only reduces fine lines and wrinkles, but it also delays the aging process.

- Treats psoriasis and eczema

One of aloe vera's greatest benefits is its ability to moisturize and hydrate skin. Eczema patients often experience dry skin that is itchy and dry. Aloe vera moisturizes their skin, relieves their itching, and calms their inflammation.

2. Rosewater

Rosewater has been long used in beauty treatments due to its powerful anti-inflammatory properties, hydrating properties, and antioxidant properties. It is highly effective both as an astringent and as an antibacterial agent, which is why it makes a great toner for absorbing dirt, oil, makeup, and anything else that might sneak into your pores.

Rosewater also offers hydrating and soothing effects, especially for people with dry, sensitive skin or for those with acne, eczema, or rosacea. Even the smell of rose reportedly diminishes the skin's sensitivity to environmental stress.

Moreover, it is an antibacterial and antioxidant, so it protects the skin from damage. Due to its high vitamin C content, rosewater may also strengthen collagen and elastin synthesis, enhancing your anti-aging routine.

3. Castile Soap

This is what provides your face wash with its cleansing properties. Castile soap is gentle and natural, and it doesn't strip the skin of its moisture, which is why it is favorable.

4. Rosehip Essential Oil

- Moisturizes your skin

Since rosehip essential oil is an emollient, it is highly effective in keeping your skin moisturized, smooth, and soft. Due to its unique balance of omega-3, omega-6, and omega-9 fatty acids, it is ideal for dehydrated and dry skin.

- Repairs skin damage

Think of your skin barrier as brick and mortar, and rosehip oil as a repairing agent that fixes any cracks and reverses the damage that lets moisture out. Fatty acids are to thank for that.

- Improves skin texture and evens skin tone

Rosehip oil is packed with antioxidants that help even out skin tone and texture. While vitamin C is best known for its ability to fade acne scars and dark spots, it is also helpful in smoothing out wrinkles and fine lines.

- Protects skin from free radicals

A number of environmental factors, including pollution and UV rays, accelerate the aging process of the skin and result in wrinkles and loss of firmness. Those free radicals are neutralized by rosehip oil, a natural antioxidant that protects the skin from the effects of free radicals.

- Provides anti-aging benefits

The anti-aging benefits of vitamins A and C include stimulating collagen production. They're great for reducing wrinkles, particularly around the eyes. Lycopene, another ingredient in the oil, is also known to be skin-rejuvenating.

- Brightens skin

You can use rosehip oil to brighten your skin. You can improve your complexion with it since it is particularly effective at treating dark spots. The oil tightens pores and brightens skin due to its astringent properties.

- Helps firm skin

If you have sagging skin, rosehip oil may help. Using it helps to achieve fresh, younger-looking skin.

5. Lavender Essential Oil

- Helps soothe dry skin

Lavender essential oil is known to maintain the oil balance of your skin. It helps in regulating the moisture barrier so that your skin neither feels too dry nor too oily. This property also makes it effective in treating several skin disorders.

- Treats scars and lightens hyperpigmentation

Its anti-inflammatory properties make lavender essential oil an excellent choice for treating inflammation. It's great for treating age spots and acne scars, plus it brightens and lightens your skin. As an antioxidant, it also helps to repair skin damage due to hyperpigmentation and scarring.

- Repairs aging skin and treats wrinkles and fine lines

The antioxidant properties of lavender essential oil help target free radicals that lead to oxidative damage. Hence, it helps to repair and protect your skin. Besides being a powerful antioxidant, lavender essential oil also stimulates collagen production. Since it has anti-aging properties, it can tighten sagging skin, as well as diminish fine lines and wrinkles.

- Calms and soothes rosacea, redness, and psoriasis

As far as healing burns, cuts, and other skin conditions are concerned, lavender essential oil is the best remedy. Lavender essential oil is antifungal, antibacterial, anti-inflammatory, and detoxifying, making it great at soothing rosacea, redness, and psoriasis. It is also suitable for treating minor cuts and scrapes.

Both psoriasis and rosacea benefit from lavender essential oil's calming and inflammation-fighting properties. Psoriasis outbreaks can also be triggered by stress, so lavender essential oil can help reduce it and promote new skin growth.

- Reduces the effects of free radicals on the skin

Lavender is known for its anti-inflammatory, anti-oxidative, and analgesic properties. By using this essential oil, oxidative damage caused by free radicals can be neutralized by the high level of anti-oxidative activity.

Hence, it also helps in promoting glowing, radiant skin.

6. Argan Oil

- Helps moisturize skin

Argan oil is beneficial for all the hydration of all skin types, but dry skin will benefit the most from this wonderful ingredient. It is light-weight, which is why it gets absorbed into your skin easily. It nour-ishes, hydrates, and moisturizes your skin for a long time.

- Prevents the transepidermal water loss

Argan oil is known to heal and seal the outer layer of your skin, contributing to not only an improved appearance, but also preventing any further damage and drying.

Essentially, it prevents transepidermal water loss, which is moisture that escapes the skin and evaporates, caused by disruptions in the outermost layer of the skin.

- Contains antioxidants

The antioxidants in argan oil help prevent environmental damage. It has anti-aging and skin-softening properties due to its high vitamin E content.

- Protects skin from sun damage

The antioxidants found in argan oil protect and repair sunburned, damaged, and hyperpigmented skin. Melanin production is inhib-ited by a number of components in argan oil.

- Has anti-inflammatory properties

Itchy and inflamed patches are characteristics of some skin condi-tions caused by dehydration. Fats like oleic and linoleic acids also have anti-inflammatory properties. Having a high content of fatty acids, argan oil locks in moisture, soothes irritated skin, and maintains your skin's barrier function.

- Abundant in fatty acids

Argan oil has a high concentration of fatty acids, which make up about 95% of its components. These fatty acids contribute to providing your skin with needed nourishment and moisturization.

2. Sandalwood and Myrrh Moisturizing Cleanser

The coconut oil in this cleanser locks in moisture and prevents your skin from drying out. It also contains sandalwood essential oil and myrrh essential oil, which are ideal oils for keeping dry skin healthy and glowing.

Ingredients Needed:

- ¾ cup distilled water
- ¼ cup liquid Castile soap
- ½ teaspoon organic coconut oil
- 3-4 drops of vitamin E oil (optional)
- 8 drops of sandalwood essential oil
- 8 drops of myrrh essential oil
- 4-6 ounce foaming soap bottle

Instructions:

1. Take the bottle and combine coconut oil, vitamin E oil, and liquid Castile soap.
2. Add in the sandalwood and myrrh essential oils.
3. Add water to the bottle until full.
4. Shake it well.
5. The cleanser is ready to be used.

How to Use the Cleanser:

1. Shake the bottle every time you want to use the cleanser.
2. Wet your face with lukewarm water.
3. Take about 2-3 pumps of the cleanser in your palm and create a lather.
4. Massage it on your face in circular motions for about a minute.
5. Rinse your face with warm water.

Benefits of Ingredients Used:

1. Coconut Oil

There are three fatty acids in coconut oil—caprylic, capric, and lauric— are antimicrobial and disinfectant. These protect against and heal microbial infections.

Various studies indicate its effectiveness in treating skin infections caused by bacteria. Research has proven that virgin coconut oil soothes and moisturizes the skin, and it's anti-inflammatory and rich in antioxidants.

- Helps soothe irritated skin

If your skin is prone to sensitivity, redness, or irritations, coconut oil helps reduce any discomfort and soothes your skin.

- Treats redness

Coconut oil helps calm temporary redness due to its calming and soothing effect.

- Adds hydration

Coconut oil consists of medium-chain fatty acids that help alleviate dryness and retain moisture levels in your skin.

- Improves skin texture

Applying coconut oil to your skin immediately makes it soft and smooth, which, as a result, improves its texture over time.

- Minimizes fine lines and wrinkles

Coconut oil aids in reducing the early signs of aging when it gets absorbed by the skin. It makes wrinkles and fine lines appear less obvious.

- Protects the skin

By forming a protective barrier on your skin, coconut oil helps shield your skin from dirt, environmental toxins, and other factors that your skin is exposed to on an everyday basis.

- Gets absorbed easily

While this may not sound like an obvious benefit, oily-skinned people benefit from this the most. While most oils are not easily absorbed into your skin, coconut oil gets absorbed fast and provides instant hydration.

2. Vitamin E Oil

- Nourishes your skin

Vitamin E oil is a great ingredient to nourish your skin. It increases blood circulation to the skin, which stimulates nourishment.

- Moisturizes your skin

Since vitamin E oil is a fat-soluble vitamin, it is heavier than the other water-soluble components. This property helps keep your skin moisturized and prevents dryness.

- Prevents early signs of aging

People with dry skin experience more fine lines and wrinkles. The antioxidants present in vitamin E help improve the blood supply to the skin, thereby preventing early skin aging. Since the oil also comes with moisturizing properties, it helps your skin look youthful and firm.

- Relieves various dry skin conditions

The anti-inflammatory property, combined with the antioxidants in vitamin E, helps relieve several dry skin conditions such as eczema, dermatitis, and psoriasis.

The oil delivers extra nourishment and prevents skin from drying, making it smooth and soft.

- Eliminates dark spots

The skin pigment melanin is responsible for dark spots or hyperpigmentation. Vitamin E oil helps treat this by reducing irritation and dryness.

- Protects from sunburns

Vitamin E oil has proven to be effective against sunburn. If your skin is sunburned, applying the oil to the affected areas will help in soothing and reducing redness. It also prevents further sun damage.

3. Sandalwood Essential Oil

Sandalwood essential oil is well known for having powerful medicinal and therapeutic properties and is a very popular aromatherapy oil. It has many different benefits for your skin.

- Hydrates your skin

Sandalwood essential oil is the perfect remedy if your skin is on the drier side, as it can replenish your epidermis to the fullest. It penetrates deeply into the skin to deliver a powerful dose of moisture as an emollient.

- Rejuvenates your skin

With its gentle astringent properties, sandalwood essential oil is the perfect ingredient for gently toning and diminishing the visible signs of aging.

- Soothes your skin

Due to its calming property, sandalwood essential oil has become increasingly popular for its rejuvenating ability. Whatever the condition is, whether it's eczema, acne, redness, or pigmentation, sandalwood has the ability to even out your skin tone and soothe your skin.

4. Myrrh Essential Oil

Myrrh essential oil is known to support healthy skin. It helps restore smooth skin and leaves it glowing and soft. Since myrrh essential oil is abundant in antioxidants and has moisturizing properties, it helps keep your skin healthy and protected. Myrrh essential oil comes to your skin's rescue if your skin is aging, dry, or chapped.

3. Honey and Olive Oil Healing Cleanser

This cleanser contains olive oil and honey, two of the most potent ingredients for dry skin. It's pretty simple to make, and all you need is 4 ingredients. The cleanser is rich in antioxidants and vitamin E, which helps in healing any skin damage, boosting collagen synthesis, and smoothing out wrinkles.

Ingredients Needed:

- 1 teaspoon liquid Castile soap
- 2 tablespoons water
- 2 tablespoons honey
- ½ cup olive oil
- A clean jar with a tight-fitting lid

Instructions:

1. Combine all the ingredients, either in a blender or with your hands, until you get a smooth and creamy consistency.
2. Pour the mixture into the jar and close it tightly.
3. Your cleanser is ready to be used.

How to Use the Cleanser:

1. Wet your face and take a small quantity of the cleanser in your palms.
2. Massage it between your hands to create a lather.
3. Gently massage your face.
4. Rinse well with water and pat your skin dry.

Benefits of Ingredients Used:

1. Honey

For thousands of years, people have used this golden goodness to promote healing and combat infection. Honey is nature's ultimate powerhouse, a fact that modern science is finally starting to confirm. It is abundant in vitamins and minerals that provide antibacterial, anti-inflammatory, and antiviral properties.

Interestingly, honey is acidic, which hinders bacterial growth, and can rid the skin of bacteria by releasing hydrogen peroxide—so those pesky bugs won't survive.

Many nutrients in honey aid in the repair and renewal of the skin. The antioxidants and essential amino acids present in honey help to improve skin elasticity, thereby reducing the signs of aging. Additionally, it can diminish the appearance of pores, which can appear on skin that is dehydrated or that has been exposed to the sun.

Honey serves as a humectant, drawing moisture into the skin, and making it more supple and firm. The second benefit of honey is its exfoliating properties, which leave your skin looking youthful and radiant. Because honey has renowned antimicrobial and anti-inflammatory properties, it may also help reduce inflammation and reduce skin redness.

2. Olive Oil

- Keeps your skin moisturized without clogging the pores

A high omega-3 and polyphenol content make olive oil one of the world's most nourishing oils. For decades, it's been a mainstay in natural beauty circles because it deeply hydrates your skin. Olive oil moisturizes the skin without clogging pores, thanks to its unique ability to mix with water.

- Maintains a youthful glow

Olive oil is a powerful natural ingredient for maintaining healthy-looking skin. The light and silky texture of olive oil make it perfect for daily moisturizing. It softens and nourishes most types of skin, giving them a subtle, natural glow.

- Balances your skin's moisture levels and protects it

Olive oil keeps your skin moisturized and prevents irritation. Oils that are oxidized can cause blackheads, but olive oil is a perfect barrier against skin irritation since it oxidizes slower than the natural oils on your skin.

- Packed with skin-beneficial nutrients

Vitamin K and squalene in olive oil, along with its antioxidants and fatty acids, contribute to skin rejuvenation and softening.

It is a natural antimicrobial, anti-inflammatory, and antibacterial agent, and has shown promising results by offering the most skin benefits.

- Has anti-aging properties

Olive oil is perfect for dealing with dry skin, which is prone to early aging signs. The anti-aging properties of this oil reduce wrinkles, fine lines, and other signs of early aging. The antioxidants in olive oil help fight free radicals. It also keeps the skin's texture firm and helps maintain its elasticity.

- Acts as an excellent exfoliator

The antioxidants present in the oil help deep clean your pores and skin. It aids in removing dead skin cells, excess oil, and dirt and leaves your skin feeling soft, fresh, and glowing. And if you are dealing with acne marks, olive oil helps tackle them as well.

- Rejuvenates your skin

Olive oil helps to rejuvenate dull, dry, and tired-looking skin. It improves blood circulation to your face, giving it the needed hydration and nourishment.

- Cleanses your skin

Olive oil effectively gets rid of dirt on the skin. Since it contains vitamin E, it is great for keeping your skin clear.

NATURAL TONER RECIPES

1. Cucumber, Aloe Vera, and Vitamin E Moisturizing Toner

This easy-to-make toner contains cucumber, aloe vera, and vitamin E, which provide your skin with intense hydration and moisturization.

Cucumber is known to be a moisturizing agent that hydrates, soothes irritation, and relieves dry, sensitive skin.

Aloe vera is known for its anti-inflammatory and hydration properties, which also aid in soothing irritated skin.

The vitamin E content in this toner helps to keep your skin smooth and soft while also providing moisturization.

Ingredients Needed:

- 1 cucumber
- 1 tablespoon aloe vera juice
- 1 vitamin E capsule
- Distilled water
- Small spritzer bottle

Instructions:

1. Wash and peel the cucumber.
2. Next, finely chop it and transfer it to a pan
3. Cover the cucumber with distilled water and heat at a low temperature for about 3-4 minutes.
4. Let it cool down.
5. Blend it, strain it, and transfer it to the spritzer bottle.
6. Add in the aloe vera juice.
7. Take the vitamin E capsule, puncture it, and add it to the mixture.
8. Mix all the ingredients well.

9. Shake the bottle each time before use.
10. Store it in the refrigerator.

Notes:

- Make sure to store this toner in the refrigerator to keep the cucumber fresh.
- Don't make this toner in bulk and use it within 4-5 days.
- Make a fresh batch after 5 days.

How To Use The Toner:

Store your toner in a spritzer bottle in the fridge and spray it directly onto your skin. When you are ready to apply it, you should:

1. Make sure your skin is clean. Remove dirt, grime, and makeup with a soap-based or oil-based cleanser. You can refer to the previous chapter to make your own cleanser with your favorite ingredients.
2. Wash your face first. Close your eyes and lightly mist it onto your face.
3. Follow it up with a serum and a moisturizer. Before applying any other skincare products, let the toner sink in for a few minutes.
4. Use this toner every morning and evening. However, if you notice any irritation or dryness, do not use toner more than once a day.

Benefits Of Ingredients Used:

1. Cucumber

- Helps hydrate your skin

The hydrating properties of cucumbers enhance skin firmness and elasticity. When our skin lacks hydration, we can visibly see the dryness and flakiness, which leads to fine lines and wrinkles. The polysaccharides in cucumbers help keep the skin moist. A cucumber contains 96% water, which allows the skin to remain hydrated.

- Treats dull skin and reduces dark circles

Several factors affect our skin, including dirt, pollution, and stress, all of which contribute to dull, dry skin. The hydrating and anti-inflammatory properties of cucumber rejuvenate and revitalize dull and lifeless skin from within.

- Reduces inflammation on the skin

The anti-inflammatory properties of cucumber are well known. Using it can help treat puffy eyes, wounds, and cuts. When you use this toner regularly, the cucumber will gradually reduce overall skin inflammation.

- Maintains your skin's overall health

Cucumbers are rich in vitamins and nutrients that maintain your skin's overall health. Cucumbers also contain antioxidants that help fight against oxidative damage from free radicals.

- Relieves sunburn

Cucumber has cooling properties that help relieve your skin from sunburn. It soothes mildly burnt and damaged skin.

- Prevents premature aging

Antioxidants in cucumbers have been shown to be highly effective in preventing wrinkles. Furthermore, cucumbers are rich in both vitamin C and folic acid. Vitamin C enables the growth of new cells, while folic acid protects against environmental toxins, which can prematurely age the skin. In combination, these components improve the firmness and health of your skin.

- Protects against free radical damage

Radiation from UV rays and pollution produce free radicals, which are unstable molecules. Your skin cells are susceptible to severe damage and your DNA is severely affected by free radicals. It has also been proven that free radicals cause skin cancer. The antioxidants in cucumbers help combat free radical damage.

- Helps tighten skin

Cucumbers have astringent properties that help in skin tightening. Cucumbers also help to close your open pores.

2. Apple Cider Vinegar and Myrrh Toner for Glowing Skin

This toner helps restore the pH levels of your skin, even out your skin tone, and keep it soft and glowing. It also helps to get rid of dead skin cells, so it promotes clear, healthy skin.

Ingredients Needed:

- ⅓ cup apple cider vinegar
- ⅔ cup witch hazel
- 3 drops of myrrh essential oil
- 4-ounce glass spray bottle

Instructions:

1. Fill a glass spray bottle with all of the ingredients.
2. Be sure to secure the lid and shake it well.
3. Always shake before using.
4. Make sure the container is airtight and not exposed to direct sunlight.

How to Use the Toner:

1. Spritz the facial toner onto your face and massage it in with a clean cloth or hand.
2. Alternatively, dampen a cotton round with toner and gently massage it into your skin.
3. It can be applied to the chest, neck, and entire face.
4. Make sure you don't get the toner in your nose, eyes, or ears.

Benefits of Ingredients Used:

1. Apple Cider Vinegar

- Gently exfoliates skin

The natural exfoliating properties of apple cider vinegar (ACV) can help you get rid of dead skin cells. The results will be glowing, youthful skin that won't show signs of aging.

- Provides relief from sunburn

ACV is an excellent treatment for sunburned and inflamed skin, since it contains anti-inflammatory properties.

- Maintains your skin's pH balance

ACV helps restore your skin's natural pH balance since it wards off pollution, bacteria, dirt, and other environmental stressors.

- Helps brighten skin

Incorporating ACV in your toner helps tighten your pores, brightens your skin, and allows other skincare products to be absorbed more easily.

2. Witch Hazel

Almost any store-bought toner contains witch hazel (and numerous homemade versions do, too). Witch hazel belongs to a family of flowering plants that grow in North America and Japan called Hamamelidaceae. It is native to these regions and has some impressive medical properties.

Some alcohol-based toners permanently strip your skin of its natural oils, but witch hazel is gentler.

- Relieves skin irritations

The tannins in witch hazel are known to reduce skin irritation. According to the Skin Protectant Monograph of the Food and Drug Administration, witch hazel is an astringent used for treating insect bites, scrapes, and minor cuts.

- Soothes skin inflammation

Witch hazel contains powerful antioxidants in the form of tannins. They reduce the effects of free radicals that are caused by environmental pollutants, thereby reducing inflammation.

- Enhances the appearance of the skin

The various benefits of witch hazel, including reducing inflammation, minimizing pores, and improving skin elasticity visibly enhance your skin's appearance.

NATURAL SERUM RECIPES

1. Lavender and Geranium Oil Serum for Dryness

This serum is packed with nutrients and helps improve your dry skin. Its main ingredients are sweet almond oil and rosehip seed oil, which keep your skin moisturized and hydrated throughout the day.

Ingredients Needed:

- 2 ½ teaspoons sweet almond oil
- 1 teaspoon rosehip seed oil
- 5 drops of lavender essential oil
- 5 drops of geranium essential oil
- 1 roller or dropper bottle

Instructions:

1. Take the dropper bottle or roller and pour the sweet almond oil and rosehip seed oil into it. You can use a mini funnel to avoid spillage.
2. Then, add 5 drops each of lavender and geranium essential oils.
3. Place the cap/roller on the bottle and shake well to combine the ingredients.
4. Store this bottle in a cool and dark place.

How to Use the Serum:

1. Cleanse your face thoroughly, ideally using a cleanser from chapter 5.
2. Then, using a cotton round or directly spraying on your face, apply a toner.
3. Next, take about 2-3 drops of the serum on your palm. Rub your palms together and gently pat your skin.
4. Massage your skin in circular motions using your fingertips.

5. Follow it with moisturizer and sunscreen during the day. Skip the sunscreen in your nighttime skincare routine.

Benefits of Ingredients Used:

1. Sweet Almond Oil

Sweet almond oil is nutrient-rich and contains the natural goodness of proteins, vitamin A, vitamin E, potassium, zinc, and essential fatty acids.

- Moisturizes skin

Almond is known as the "king of nuts" for good reason, sweet almond oil helps keep your skin beautiful.

Wrinkles and age spots are sometimes indicative of our age, as they occur because of harsh environmental factors, stress, and aging. As a rich source of vitamin E, almond oil is beneficial for maintaining healthy skin.

- Maintains a youthful and healthy complexion

An even layer of padding under your skin is provided by collagen, the protein responsible for maintaining your skin's youth. Skin thins with age, and collagen padding beneath becomes uneven, causing fine lines and wrinkles to appear. Sweet almond oil contains vitamin E, which can support collagen growth. Over time, this will promote skin health, and your skin will remain even and healthy.

- Protects your skin from damage

The vitamin E in sweet almond oil keeps your skin supple, smooth, and wrinkle-free by protecting it from UV rays.

- Soothes and heals chapped, irritated skin

Sweet almond oil contains fatty acids that help in healing and soothing irritated, chapped skin and retaining moisture.

- Helps soothe puffy eyes

Sweet almond oil is an anti-inflammatory, which eases the swelling of the skin under your eyes.

- Heals dry skin

If your skin is scratchy, flaky, and itchy, sweet almond oil will be your savior! The fatty acids present in the oil help retain moisture and keep your skin hydrated.

2. Geranium Essential Oil

Geranium oil acts as an astringent to help minimize wrinkles and fine lines by tightening your skin and slowing down the effects of aging. Geranium oil also prevents bacteria from growing on your skin due to its powerful cicatrizant properties, which help to increase the blood flow under the surface of your skin. The oil is also beneficial in speeding up the healing process and will fade scars faster.

2. Avocado and Frankincense Oil Anti-Aging Serum

Ingredients Needed:

- 2 tablespoons avocado oil
- 2 tablespoons rosewater
- 2 teaspoons aloe vera gel
- 3-5 drops of vitamin E oil
- 3 drops of frankincense essential oil
- A glass bottle with a dropper

Instructions:

1. Combine rosewater with aloe vera gel in a bowl. Stir well so that no lumps remain.
2. Next, add vitamin E oil and frankincense essential oil. Gently stir the mixture to combine the ingredients.
3. After all the ingredients are completely dissolved and well mixed, pour the serum into a clean glass bottle and refrigerate for one day. After that, it's ready to use.
4. Shake it well before each use.

How to Use the Serum:

1. To use the serum, take 3-4 drops on your palm.
2. Apply it all over your face and neck.

Benefits Of Ingredients Used:

1. Avocado Oil

- Moisturizes and nourishes your skin

Avocado oil is rich in minerals, lipids, vitamin A, vitamin C, vitamin D, and vitamin E, which nourish your skin. It hydrates and soothes chapped, damaged, and dry skin. This oil contributes to the restoration of the skin barrier by enhancing its permeability. Therefore, avocado oil may improve skincare product absorption.

- Soothes sun-damaged skin

Avocado oil soothes inflammation and UV-damaged skin. Avocado oil contains polyhydroxylated fatty alcohols (PFA) that reduce inflammation and damage caused by UV rays. In addition, avocado oil can be applied to soothe sunburns and prevent skin aging, dark spots, and pigmentation.

- Promotes wound healing and development of collagen

Avocado oil contains vitamins and fatty acids that help heal wounds and develop collagen, thereby improving the tensile strength of your skin. This keeps your skin bouncy and youthful.

- Reduces inflammation

Avocado oil possessesanti-inflammatory properties and helps reduce skin inflammation.

- Has anti-aging properties

Pigmentation, fine lines, wrinkles, and dark spots on the skin can be treated with avocado oil due to its anti-inflammatory and UV-protective properties. Using avocado oil can rejuvenate the dermis, which keeps the skin strong and flexible.

2. *Frankincense Essential Oil*

In the world of essential oils, frankincense is known as the "king" of them all!

- Helps moisturize and balance skin

As a moisturizing agent, frankincense essential oil protects the skin against dryness.

- Contains anti-aging properties

The anti-aging properties come from frankincense's powerful antioxidant content.

- Combats free radical damage

Free radicals are known as highly reactive molecules carrying unpaired electrons, which can be combated with antioxidants. DNA is damaged when these free radicals move throughout the body in search of electrons, which accelerates aging. Antioxidants present in the oil slow down and stop free radical damage. It thus helps rejuvenate the skin.

- Has astringent properties

Frankincense essential oil has astringent properties. It helps heal skin imperfections and skin conditions such as acne and wounds. Historically, frankincense oil has been used as a healing oil for restoring damaged skin. You can also use this oil to reduce scars and stretch marks.

- Provides skin protection

Frankincense oil's antiseptic, antibacterial, and antioxidant properties reduce inflammation, protect the skin from damage, and negate free radical effects.

NATURAL EYE CREAM RECIPES

1. Eye Cream for Wrinkles, Dark Circles, and Puffiness

Collagen production decreases with age. Dark circles and puffiness under the eyes can also occur due to stress and lack of sleep. For people with puffy eyes, dark circles, and perhaps even wrinkles, this eye cream works wonders. By helping to reduce puffiness and tighten the skin around your eyes, it is a kind of anti-aging lotion.

For making this effective under-eye cream, you only need a few ingredients. The main one is coconut oil. Vitamin E oil and some essential oils are also used.

Ingredients Needed:

- ⅛ cup coconut oil
- 10 drops of vitamin E oil
- 10 drops of frankincense essential oil
- 10 drops of lavender essential oil
- 10 drops of cypress essential oil
- A mason jar with a lid

Instructions:

1. Add all the ingredients to a mixing bowl and combine well.
2. To store, transfer into an airtight container, such as a mason jar with a lid.

Note:

- You can keep this eye cream in the fridge or at room temperature below 76 degrees Fahrenheit.

How to Use the Eye Cream:

1. Apply this eye cream on your eyelids, around the eye area, and under the eyes. Then massage it gently into your skin.
2. Apply it daily before going to bed, preferably after washing your face and applying moisturizer.

Benefits of Ingredients Used

1. Coconut Oil

Since coconut oil helps keep connective tissue strong, it is a great ingredient for eye cream. The skin around the eyes may appear smoother, and fine lines and wrinkles may disappear. Coconut oil has antibacterial, antifungal, and moisturizing properties that are beneficial to dry skin. It is also extremely gentle on sensitive areas such as the eyelids and the face.

2. Vitamin E Oil

Vitamin E oil helps slow down the aging process. When used in an under-eye cream, vitamin E oil provides the same benefits as coconut oil, since it has a mild consistency that is suitable for sensitive skin.

3. Frankincense Essential Oil

Using frankincense essential oil reduces the appearance of age spots, sun spots, and discoloration of the skin. Use frankincense essential oil to help even out uneven skin tone and prevent dark circles under your eyes. Additionally, it works well for tightening and improving your skin's texture.

4. Lavender Essential Oil

Lavender essential oil is known to reduce signs of skin imperfections and has many other amazing properties. This is a great essential oil to use on the face because it is very gentle.

Lavender essential oil is an antiseptic and anti-inflammatory that helps to fight bacteria causing inflammation and acne. It is also a powerful antioxidant that controls sebum and detoxifies the skin.

Lavender soothes occasional skin irritations and disperses the appearance of skin imperfections. Moreover, it is effective for reducing the appearance of scars, blemishes, bumps, and rashes. Since lavender essential oil is very gentle and can be used on sensitive skin, it is great to use on the face and under the eyes.

5. Cypress Essential Oil

Cypress oil is great for treating dark circles under the eyes, as it increases blood circulation when applied topically to the skin.

2. Coffee-Infused Eye Cream for Fine Lines

Caffeine is proven to have a wide range of health benefits, ranging from boosting physical alertness and treating migraines to improving memory and maintaining a healthy heart. It can also do wonders for the skin!

Caffeine can reduce dark circles under the eyes, reduce puffiness, tighten skin, and fight free radicals. It's very common for eye creams to contain coffee due to its amazing benefits. Here's an easy recipe to make your own coffee-infused eye cream.

Ingredients Needed:

- ¼ cup beeswax
- ¼ cup coconut oil
- ¼ cup coffee-infused oil
- 1 teaspoon jojoba oil
- 4-5 drops of chamomile essential oil
- 3 capsules of vitamin E
- A metal tin or a mason jar with a lid
- A double boiler (or a heat-proof container)

Instructions:

1. Take the beeswax and place it in a glass bowl, then place the bowl in water on low heat. Once the beeswax has melted, add the coconut oil, jojoba oil, coffee-infused oil, and vitamin E oil, stirring after each addition.
2. Take the pot off the heat and stir in 4 to 5 drops of chamomile essential oil. You want every drop to be filled with caffeine goodness, so make sure you mix it thoroughly!
3. Transfer to a tin container or a storage container. Refrigerate to solidify.

Note:

- You can expect your eye cream to last up to a year.

How to Use the Eye Cream:

1. Use this caffeine-infused eye cream twice a day after you've freshly cleansed your face. Apply an appropriate amount to the under-eye area and allow it to seep in thoroughly (you don't have to rinse it off).
2. You can apply a cold dab of this eye cream and give the under-eye area a massage using a jade roller on your face if you feel your face is puffier than usual.
3. You could also use a jade gua sha if you don't to promote lymphatic drainage on your face. Gua sha complements this cream's rich texture, leaving you with a perfectly rejuvenated under-eye area.

Benefits of Ingredients Used:

1. Coffee

Caffeine is the primary compound in coffee—the part of the beverage that we are familiar with and love. Since caffeine is an antioxidant, it offers protection against sun damage and free radicals that lead to wrinkles.

Furthermore, caffeine acts as a vasoconstrictor, meaning that when ingested or applied topically to specific areas, it constricts the blood vessels. These constricting effects may help reduce puffiness under the eyes, reduce redness, and reduce the appearance of dark circles by reducing swelling.

With all the antioxidants present in coffee, you can prevent premature aging and achieve that smooth complexion you've always wanted. Coffee also removes cellulite, so you can use it on other areas of your body as well!

2. Beeswax

Besides thickening the eye cream, beeswax also has skin-benefiting properties. Beeswax is an anti-inflammatory, which is beneficial for puffy or swollen eyes. Additionally, beeswax is a rich source of vitamin A. Beeswax seals in moisture and is an excellent ingredient for eye creams, as it gives you an extra boost of hydration.

NATURAL MOISTURIZER RECIPES

1. Aloe Vera and Beeswax Soothing Moisturizer

Aloe vera is a boon for people with extremely dry, irritated skin. This recipe also contains beeswax, which helps create a protective layer on your skin. It is also known to be a humectant, meaning that it attracts water from the environment. These qualities of both aloe vera and beeswax help in keeping your skin hydrated for longer.

Ingredients Needed:

- ½ cup aloe vera gel
- 50 ml coconut oil
- 50 ml almond oil
- 10 tablespoon beeswax
- 3-5 drops of chamomile essential oil
- 3-5 drops of lavender essential oil

Instructions:

1. Melt coconut oil, almond oil, and beeswax together using either a double boiler or double-boiling method.
2. Once this mixture cools down, add aloe vera, chamomile, and lavender essential oils.
3. Blend this concoction until you get a creamy consistency.
4. Store it in an airtight jar.

How To Use The Moisturizer:

Use this moisturizer just like any other moisturizer.

1. Clean your face and follow it up with a toner, serum, and eye cream.
2. Take a pea-sized amount of moisturizer on your fingers.
3. Apply it to your skin and massage it until it is absorbed.

4. Follow it up with sunscreen during the day.
5. Use it twice daily.

Benefits Of Ingredients Used:

1. Beeswax

- Forms a natural barrier on your skin

Beeswax tends to form a natural protective barrier on your skin's surface which helps prevent water loss and keeps your skin soft, nourished, and hydrated. This barrier also protects your skin from harmful environmental irritants.

For acne-prone skin, beeswax is especially helpful because it keeps pores unblocked, allowing them to breathe.

- Softens and moisturizes skin

Since beeswax is softening and lubricating, it helps reduce transepidermal water loss.

- Improves elasticity

Beeswax contains ingredients that contribute to soft skin, thereby improving the elasticity of your skin. It also helps improve the texture of your skin by retaining moisture.

- Has antibacterial and antiseptic properties

Beeswax is rich in squalene, flavonoids, and 10-hydroxy-trans-2-decanoic acid, which comes with antibacterial and antiseptic properties. Hence, it helps to protect your skin against microorganisms and pathogens.

- Soothes skin

Beeswax helps soothe your skin since it is antioxidant, anti-inflammatory, and anti-allergenic in nature. This makes it an ideal ingredient for not only people with dry skin, but also for people with sensitive skin.

- Has anti-aging effects

Beeswax also contains β-carotene, a rich source of vitamin A. This helps stimulate the mitotic cell division in your epidermis and delays the degradation of collagen. This, in turn, leads to faster cell regeneration.

2. Chamomile Essential Oil

Chamomile essential oil is an excellent ingredient for soothing your skin due to its powerful anti-inflammatory and calming properties. You can use chamomile essential oil to soothe itchy skin, reduce breakouts, and re-ignite your skin's radiance.

This oil can also relieve dry skin-related conditions such as eczema and psoriasis.

Chamomile oil has many benefits:

- Moisturizer
- Effective treatment for skin conditions like eczema
- Treating inflammation and redness of the skin
- Relieve itching and skin irritation caused by skin allergies
- Even out your skin tone when applied regularly
- Repair and regenerate the skin, resulting in a fresh, youthful appearance

2. Almond Oil and Cocoa Butter Moisturizer for Flaky, Itchy Skin

If you have extremely dry and flaky skin, this moisturizer will become your go-to! It contains almond oil and cocoa butter, two of the best ingredients for revitalizing and rejuvenating your skin.

If you use this moisturizer regularly, your skin will be left soft, smooth, and supple.

Ingredients:

- 1 tablespoon sweet almond oil
- 2 tablespoons cocoa butter
- 1 tablespoon aloe vera gel
- 3-4 drops of rosewater

Instructions:

1. Put almond oil and cocoa butter into a container and melt them together.
2. Add aloe vera gel and rosewater.
3. Prepare the paste by mixing together all the ingredients.
4. Store it in an airtight container.

Benefits of Ingredients Used:

1. Cocoa Butter

- Deeply moisturizes your skin

With its high fatty acid content and ability to hydrate the skin deeply, cocoa butter is the perfect ingredient for moisturizers and lip balms. It is packed with oleic, stearic, and palmitic acids. These ingredients deeply nourish and moisturize your skin.

- A powerful antioxidant

Cocoa butter contains antioxidants that protect your skin from the damage caused by free radicals, like dullness, dark patches, and aging skin. You must protect your skin from free-radical damage if you want it to stay young and healthy. The anti-inflammatory properties of cocoa butter also help your skin resist the aging process.

- Prevents the appearance of stretch marks and heals scarring

The rich moisturizing properties of cocoa butter help prevent the appearance of stretch marks. If you have scarring, cocoa butter repairs your skin by healing the marks and the damage to your skin cells.

- Heals and repairs dry, damaged skin

Cocoa butter can heal and repair damaged, dry skin—thanks to its restorative properties. It contains emollients and healthy fats, which nourish and restore the skin from deep within.

- Delays the process of aging

As a good source of fatty acids and antioxidants, cocoa butter prevents wrinkles, darkening, and dullness caused by free radicals. As a result, it prevents the signs of aging by keeping the skin hydrated and nourished.

- Reduces irritation and inflammation

Cocoa butter is perfect for itchy, red skin. Even severe skin diseases, such as eczema and psoriasis, seem to benefit from its healing properties. Cocoa butter will soothe your skin, resulting in quick relief from itching and dryness.

NATURAL FACE OIL RECIPES

1. Rosehip and Marula Oil Moisturizing Anti-Aging Oil

This is an extra-rich oil containing rosehip oil and marula oil, both of which are not only moisturizing but also anti-aging. When mixed with rose and carrot essential oils, this concoction provides your skin with nourishment and hydration. It is beneficial for people with extremely dry, flaky skin. You can use this oil on your face and as well as your neck to stay moisturized.

Ingredients Needed:

- 2 tablespoons argan oil
- 1 tablespoon marula oil
- 1 tablespoon rosehip oil
- 12 drops of rose essential oil
- 5 drops of carrot seed oil
- A dropper bottle

Instructions:

1. Add all the oils together in a dropper bottle.
2. Shake it well to mix the ingredients.

How to Use the Oil

1. Massage the oil gently into the skin in an upward motion, beginning at the jawline and working up. Avoid the area around your eyes.
2. Shake the bottle thoroughly before every use so that any oils that may have separated between applications are recombined.

Benefits of Ingredients Used:

1. Marula Oil

- Maintains moisture balance

Marula oil contains a wide range of emollients, including vitamin E, Omega-3, Omega-6, and Omega-9 fatty acids, which makes it an excellent moisturizer. It also has 78% oleic acid, which retains moisture and makes your skin soft and radiant.

- Helps balance and replenish the skin barrier

Marula oil is rich in oleic and omega acids, which help replenish and repair the skin's barrier function.

- Protects skin against harsh environmental pollutants

This oil is known to shield your skin against the harmful effects of environmental pollutants, harsh UV rays of the sun, and cold winds. It facilitates the natural renewal process of your skin while you are asleep and helps reverse the damage caused by environmental factors. In addition, it contains a combination of nourishing and moisturizing ingredients that give the skin a healthy glow from the inside out.

- Acts an occlusive

Marula oil is occlusive by nature, meaning that it creates a thin layer on your skin to seal in all the goodness and moisture. Thanks to its high fatty acid content (oleic and linoleic), it softens and nourishes your skin. Despite the high fatty acid content, it's super lightweight and won't leave you feeling greasy.

- Provides antioxidant protection

We know that for achieving soft, supple, and hydrated skin, we need antioxidants, and marula oil is a rich source of these. It is primarily packed with vitamin C, vitamin E, and epicatechin, a strong, phytochemical antioxidant. These antioxidants help keep the free radicals at bay.

- Prevents and heals skin disorders such as eczema

Skin disorders like eczema and dermatitis are characterized by one or more of the following symptoms: itching, redness, flaking, cracking or bleeding. Omega-3, 6 and 9 fatty acids along with vitamin E make marula oil an excellent topical treatment for exfoliating the skin and treating eczema.

As it moisturizes generously, it calms the oil glands that go crazy when the skin is dry. Marula's nutrients provide anti-inflammatory properties that protect against bacterial invasion and further inflammation.

- Has anti-aging properties

Marula oil consists of 4 times as much vitamin C as oranges and 60% more antioxidants than coconut oil, argan oil, and several other natural oils. It also contains vitamin E and oleic acid, a potent Omega-9 that is known to keep fine lines, wrinkles, and dryness at bay.

Antioxidants, moisture-locking ingredients, and anti-inflammatory properties work together to prevent the sagging of the skin, fight free radicals, and hydrate dull and dry skin. Moreover, Omega-9 fatty acids and other fatty acids promote collagen production and skin regeneration throughout this process.

- Improves the penetration of other skincare products

The high oleic acid content of marula oil allows other skincare products to better penetrate the skin.

2. Rose Essential Oil

- Hydrates skin

Traditionally, rose essential oil has been used for hydrating and reinforcing the skin barrier.

- Has antibacterial properties

The antibacterial properties of rose oil make it ideal for treating acne. It can both nourish and disinfect your skin. Moreover, it is powerful enough to remove scars and other imperfections.

- Reduces wrinkles

Rose oil is one of the best anti-aging essential oils. The beauty-enhancing properties of rose oil date back centuries. Its main benefit is that it keeps skin looking younger for a longer period of time.

Citronellol and geraniol are antioxidants found in rose oil that help fight free radical damage and slow the signs of aging. Free radicals harm the skin tissue and can cause fine lines, wrinkles, and dehydration.

Rose oil has natural properties that make it beneficial for all skin types, particularly mature, dry, and sensitive skin. Additionally, it treats eczema and rosacea, as well as broken capillaries and scarring.

- Has anti-inflammatory properties

Historically, rose oil has been used as an astringent and to treat inflammation. Many skin conditions can benefit from it, including eczema, sun damage, stretch marks, and scarring.

3. Carrot Seed Oil

- It slows down the aging process

As an antioxidant, carrot seed oil fights free radicals and removes aging signs. It also contains several vitamins such as vitamin A which prevents skin from aging, vitamin C which promotes collagen synthesis, and vitamin E which moisturizes the skin and minimizes wrinkles. This oil also promotes cell regeneration, making your skin supple.

- Soothing

Carrot seed oil has anti-inflammatory properties and an earthy aroma. The skin benefits from these in several ways. When applied to the face, carrot seed oil reduces inflammation, irritation, acne, and scarring caused by acne. As a result, the skin remains clear.

- Has antibacterial properties

Carrot seed oil is an effective antibacterial agent. By inhibiting the growth of harmful bacteria, it protects the skin from breakouts. There is no damage to the underlying skin from the oil because it targets only the bacteria.

- Prevents skin damage caused by the sun

This oil has also been found to be helpful in protecting the skin from the damaging effects of the sun. It has an SPF rating of 30-40, which makes it a useful UV-blocking agent.

- Has anti-inflammatory properties

The anti-inflammatory properties of carrot seed oil help soothe the scalp and skin. Using it can reduce inflammation, irritation, and acne.

- Treats a variety of skin conditions

Carrot seed oil helps in treating skin conditions like eczema, psoriasis, dermatitis, and vitiligo. Due to its antibacterial properties, it helps in inhibiting bacterial growth. It also destroys bacteria responsible for these skin conditions, helping to treat them.

2. Avocado and Apricot Seed Oil for Anti-Aging and Skin Rejuvenation

As a rich source of fatty acids, antioxidants, and vitamin E, apricot seed oil rejuvenates the skin from the inside out. It prevents blackheads and fine lines while softening and soothing the skin.

The fatty acids and oleic acid in avocado oil stimulate collagen production. The lecithin, vitamin D, and vitamin E in it prevent premature aging and soothe the skin. In addition to its anti-inflammatory properties, it moisturizes the skin deeply.

The lavender oil in this recipe hydrates and moisturizes chapped skin.

Ingredients Needed:

- 1 vitamin E capsule
- 5-6 drops of lavender oil
- 1 teaspoon avocado oil
- 1 teaspoon apricot kernel oil
- 5-6 drops of rosemary essential oil

Instructions:

1. Combine lavender essential oil, rosemary essential oil, apricot kernel oil, and avocado oil.
2. Next, add in vitamin E.
3. Mix all ingredients well.
4. Using gentle circular motions, apply this mixture to your face.

Benefits of Ingredients Used:

1. Apricot Kernel Oil

- Intensively nourishing

The apricot kernel oil contains vitamins and minerals that deeply nourish the skin. Due to the skin's porous nature, apricot oil can penetrate deep into the protective surface layers and benefits the skin long-term.

- Softens and moisturizes your skin

The light texture of apricot kernel oil allows it to penetrate deeply into the skin and moisturize it. It contains a high amount of vitamin A, which makes your skin supple and soft. It moisturizes skin that is sensitive and dry. Furthermore, it smooths the texture of your skin.

- Brings a radiant glow to your skin

Apricot oil contains vitamin E, which enhances the skin's ability to combat free radicals. It also helps to clear up blemishes. This results in radiant skin.

- Acts as a protective barrier

In order to protect the skin against oxidative damage, faster cell turnover is crucial. Apricot oil will nourish and protect your skin, no matter what your age is.

- Has anti-inflammatory properties

Apricot oil is extremely nourishing, which means that it can reduce the severity of skin conditions such as acne, rosacea, and psoriasis. When you have a flare-up, using apricot oil will aid in stress relief and promote healthier skin.

• Prevents early signs of aging

This oil helps nourish the skin. Consequently, it minimizes fine lines, wrinkles, and other signs of aging. It is rich in vitamin A, which promotes cell turnover on your face. As a result, the youngest cells appear on the surface, giving the skin a more youthful look.

Additionally, vitamin A helps plump the skin by supporting the skin cells. It reduces the appearance of wrinkles and fine lines.

• Protects your skin from harmful UV rays

Due to its antioxidant properties, it provides protection against free radicals and harmful rays. The result is even-toned, smooth skin.

2. Rosemary essential Oil

• Protects against free radicals

Rosemary essential oil is rich in antioxidants that promote healthy skin by protecting it against free radicals.

• Has anti-inflammatory properties

Rosemary oil contains terpenes that calm and soothe irritated skin.

• Treats acne

The antimicrobial and antifungal properties of rosemary essential oil help reduce the appearance of blemishes and control acne breakouts.

• Regulates production of sebum

Rosemary oil helps to balance sebum production, making it ideal for oily skin types.

- Helps improve skin texture

The astringent properties of rosemary oil help to improve the tonicity and texture of the skin.

- Helps reduce puffiness

Rosemary oil helps to enhance blood circulation, which reduces fluid retention and puffiness. It also helps to promote an even skin tone.

NATURAL SUNSCREEN RECIPE

Protect your skin from harmful UVA and UVB rays with this natural sunscreen recipe. It is extremely easy to make and use. This sunscreen is also waterproof, thanks to beeswax. It forms a barrier on your skin, thereby letting the water runoff. Moreover, beeswax is rich in vitamin A, which supports the process of cell regeneration.

Ingredients Needed:

- ½ cup jojoba oil
- ¼ cup beeswax pellets
- ¼ cup non-nano zinc oxide
- ¼ cup cocoa butter
- ¼ cup coconut oil
- 15 drops of frankincense essential oil
- 15 drops of peppermint essential oil
- A mason jar with a wide mouth

Instructions:

1. Put coconut oil, beeswax, cocoa butter, and avocado oil in a double boiler and melt them together. Put the ingredients in a bowl on top of a pot of water and bring them to a boil if you don't have a double boiler.
2. Remove the bowl from the heat once the ingredients have melted completely.
3. Next, add non-nano zinc oxide.
4. Add 15 drops each of frankincense essential oil and peppermint essential oil. Whisk them well.
5. Lastly, put the sunscreen in a wide-mouthed mason jar.

Notes:

- Make sure the sunscreen is stored in an airtight glass container. If you intend to use this sunscreen at the beach or pool, make sure to store it in a plastic container.
- If using a plastic container, do not add the essential oils to the recipe. Essential oils break plastics down.
- Remember: Water and essential oils do not mix well together.
- You can store this sunscreen for up to one year. If water enters this sunscreen, then its shelf life will be drastically shortened.

Benefits of Ingredients Used:

1. Cocoa Butter

Cocoa butter smells divine and has amazing benefits. It hydrates and nourishes your skin, and also helps treat skin irritations and rashes. As a bonus, it smells heavenly when combined with peppermint essential oil!

2. Non-nano Zinc Oxide

Zinc oxide is a mineral powder that is undoubtedly one of the safest sun protectants. It offers protection against UVA and UVB rays.

Be sure to buy non-nano zinc oxide when purchasing zinc oxide. When applied to the skin, zinc oxide nanoparticles are easily absorbed into the body. Nano zinc oxide is toxic to marine life, but non-nano zinc oxide is considered marine-safe.

NATURAL LIP BALM RECIPES

1. Raspberry Tinted Lip Balm for a Flush of Color

You can make your own tinted lip balm with just three ingredients, and get that flush of color along with the nourishing benefits.

Ingredients Needed:

- 1-2 tablespoons coconut oil
- ½ tablespoonfreeze-dried raspberries
- ½-1 teaspoon beeswax

Instructions:

1. Grind the raspberries using a coffee grinder, food processor, or mortar and pestle to get a fine powder.
2. Melt beeswax and coconut oil together using a double boiler. Alternatively, you can add them to a Pyrex measuring cup and place them in a saucepan. Fill it with 2 inches of water and put it to boil at low heat.
3. Next, add the raspberry powder and mix well.
4. Transfer the mixture to a container with a lid and allow it to harden.

Notes:

- Use this lip balm within 3-6 months. If you notice a change in consistency or mold growth, discard it immediately.

Benefits of Ingredients Used:

1. Raspberries

The color of raspberries makes them great for homemade cosmetics. They're beneficial for your skin, and your lips too! In addition to vitamin C and polyphenols, raspberries are rich in antioxidants, which can help prevent premature aging of your skin by protecting it from free radical damage.

Raspberries also contain magnesium, vitamin E, lutein (a brain enhancer), and the antioxidants of beta-carotene and flavonoids.

2. Beeswax

Apart from the previously discussed benefits of beeswax, it also benefits your lips. The antiviral, anti-inflammatory, and antibacterial properties of this ingredient make it ideal for treating chapped lips or skin. Additionally, it keeps moisture sealed in your lips and prevents them from drying.

2. Rose Oil Nourishing and Protecting Lip Balm

Soothe your dry, chapped, and cracked lips with this lip balm. It contains beeswax that seals in moisture and acts as a protective barrier for your lips. It also provides a protective layer from external elements like cold weather and wind.

Ingredients Needed:

- 2 tablespoons coconut oil
- 2 tablespoons cocoa butter
- 2 tablespoons beeswax
- 10 drops of rose essential oil
- Lip balm tubes (you will be able to fill about 12 tubes with this recipe)

Instructions:

1. Put all the ingredients in a double boiler, except the rose essential oil. You can also put the ingredients in a glass bowl and place the bowl in a pot of boiling water if you don't have a double boiler.
2. Keep stirring the mixture until the ingredients are melted.

3. Remove the mixture from the heat and add rose essential oil.
4. Using a small funnel, medicine dropper, or pipette, fill the lip balm tubes. Make sure to do this step as quickly as possible before the mixture starts to harden.
5. Allow them to settle, cool, and harden completely before you cap them.

Notes:

- You can store the extra lip balm tubes in a cool and dry place.
- When stored in a cool, dry place, this lip balm has a shelf-life of more than two years.

Benefits of Ingredients Used:

1. Cocoa Butter

Apart from the benefits of cocoa butter discussed previously, the moisturizing properties of cocoa butter help heal dry, chapped skin.

2. Rose Essential Oil

In addition to the benefits discussed before and its wonderful smell, rose essential oil is ideal for treating any type of skin imperfection, including dry, cracked and aggravated skin on the lips.

NATURAL EXFOLIATOR RECIPES

1. Whipped Rose Sugar Scrub for Glowing Skin

This whipped rose sugar scrub is made with just four ingredients: brown sugar, coconut oil, rose essential oil, and vitamin E oil. It will leave your skin feeling smooth, hydrated, and rejuvenated. These ingredients remove the dead skin cells gently yet effectively and will leave your skin feeling smooth and soft.

Ingredients Needed:

- 1 cup brown sugar
- ½ cup coconut oil
- 10 drops of rose essential oil
- 5 drops of vitamin E oil

Instructions:

1. Take a hand mixer and whip coconut oil for 10 minutes. Add it to a clean mixing bowl.
2. Then add brown sugar, rose essential oil, and vitamin E oil to the bowl.
3. Continue to whip the mixture until all the ingredients are combined well.
4. Transfer the mixture to an airtight container.

How to Use the Scrub:

1. You shouldn't use sugar scrubs or any other exfoliator on a daily basis. Use this scrub a maximum of 3 times a week.
2. To remove dead skin cells, apply the scrub to cleansed skin. Gently massage it in and then let it sit for a couple of minutes.
3. After rinsing, pat the skin dry with a soft towel.

Benefits of Ingredients Used:

1. Brown Sugar

- Gentle on the skin

Salt scrubs can sometimes cause microscopic tears on your skin because of the size of the grains. The smaller particles in brown sugar make it more gentle and safer to use.

- Minimizes pores

The antibacterial properties of brown sugar prevent harmful toxins from entering the skin. The glycolic acid in it helps eliminate dead skin cells. Getting rid of buildup gives you a radiant and clear complexion. By exfoliating, these sugar granules tighten pores and prevent oil buildup.

- Enhances blood circulation

When brown sugar is massaged into the skin, it increases blood circulation, which helps to maintain a youthful appearance. Furthermore, brown sugar scrub enhances the firmness of the skin and prolongs collagen's lifespan.

- Gets rid of pigmentation

Brown sugar exfoliates the skin, making it smoother. Glycolic acid in brown sugar helps even the skin tone.

- Prevents early aging signs

Regular exfoliation enhances the appearance of the skin by promoting collagen synthesis. Brown sugar's anti-aging properties minimize wrinkles and fine lines when it is used as an exfoliant.

2. Oats and Honey Moisturizing Exfoliator

Ingredients Needed:

- ¼ cup oats
- 2 tablespoons coconut oil
- 1 teaspoon honey

Instructions:

1. Mix all three ingredients thoroughly in a bowl.
2. Store the scrub in an airtight container with a lid.

How to Use the Scrub:

1. Use clean hands to scrub damp skin.
2. Start by massaging your jaw and work your way upward, making sure to avoid the eye area.
3. Use lukewarm water to rinse.
4. Then, follow it up with a toner, serum, and moisturizer or oil.

Benefits of Ingredients Used:

1. Oats

Your skin can benefit tremendously from oats, which are great for fighting acne. The saponins in them remove dirt and oil, making them a good homemade facial cleanser. For dry skin and conditions like eczema and psoriasis, oats have great soothing and anti-inflammatory properties.

NATURAL FACE MASK RECIPES

1. Avocado and Aloe Vera Nourishing Face Mask

This face mask consists of avocado, aloe vera gel, honey, and lavender essential oil to provide your skin with deep hydration and nourishment. Coconut oil is a moisturizing agent and combined with the natural humectant honey, it helps to retain the moisture in your skin. Avocado is also packed with vitamins and antioxidants that help deliver intense nourishment from within. And lastly, aloe vera hydrates and rejuvenates your skin.

This mask is simple to make and needs just four ingredients.

Ingredients Needed:

- ¼ ripe avocado
- 2 tablespoons aloe vera gel
- 1 tablespoon honey
- 2-3 drops of lavender essential oil

Instructions:

1. Beat and mash the avocado in a bowl.
2. Add honey and aloe vera gel. Mix them well.
3. Add lavender essential oil to this mixture and stir well.
4. The mask is ready and should be used immediately.

Note:

- This recipe is for one mask. Only make this mask when you intend to use it. Discard any leftovers.

How to Use the Mask:

1. Apply a thin layer evenly over your face and neck. Make sure you leave the mask on for 15-20 minutes for maximum effectiveness. Avoid contact with the eyes, nose, and ear canals.
2. Ideally, you should apply it after washing your face. When you're finished with the mask, apply moisturizer to your face.

Benefits of Ingredients Used:

1. Avocado

- Deeply moisturizes skin

There are about 62% lipids in avocado oil, including polyunsaturated and monounsaturated fats. Compared to other popular plant oils, such as almond oil and olive oil, avocado oil penetrates the skin deeper. Avocado is therefore an excellent moisturizer, especially if you have flaky, chapped, or dry skin.

- Rich in antioxidants

Avocados contain antioxidants, such as polyphenols and carotenoids, that help prevent free radical damage. Inadequate sleep, pollution, and UV rays are some of the environmental aggressors that form these compounds. Free radicals can damage DNA in skin cells and accelerate skin aging when they accumulate on the skin. Over time, this results in wrinkles, age spots, fine lines, and other signs of aging. Avocado oil's antioxidants neutralize these damaging compounds, ensuring that the skin is healthy and protected from external stresses.

- Prevents wrinkles and delays signs of aging

Avocados are also rich in vitamin E and vitamin C, both of which play a crucial role in supporting healthier skin and preventing free radical damage. Furthermore, avocados are rich in antioxidants such as zeaxanthin and lutein, which combat free radical formation.

- Soothes skin

Avocados are packed with vitamins and healthy fats that not only repair the skin, but also improve its appearance and make it more radiant and clear.

2. Coconut and Cocoa Hydrating Mask

This mask contains three ingredients that are a boon for people with dry skin: coconut oil, cocoa powder, and honey. Coconut oil gives deep nourishment, avocado is hydrating, and cocoa is packed with skin-soothing antioxidants.

Ingredients Needed:

- 1 tablespoon coconut oil
- 1 tablespoon cocoa powder
- 1 tablespoon honey

Instructions:

1. Take a mixing bowl and mix all the ingredients together.
2. Apply this mask to clean and dry skin.
3. Leave it on for 10 minutes and wash it off with lukewarm water.
4. Follow it up with a moisturizer.

Note:

- This recipe is for one mask. Only make this mask when you intend to use it. Discard any leftovers.

Benefits of Ingredients Used:

1. Cocoa Powder

- Antioxidant powerhouse

The flavonoids in cocoa, called flavonols, are powerful antioxidants.

By repairing the damage free radicals cause, antioxidants protect your skin from harmful environmental toxins such as ultraviolet light, household chemicals, car exhaust fumes, and cigarette smoke. In addition to boosting blood flow, they promote cell growth, which keeps your skin looking youthful and radiant.

- Helps brighten skin

Cocoa powder accelerates the renewal of skin cells because of its healing properties. Cocoa powder contains theobromine, which promotes blood flow to the surface of the skin. As a result, your skin appears younger and brighter. The vitamin C content in it reduces hyperpigmentation, fades dark spots, and lightens blemishes.

- Combats signs of aging

There are many benefits associated with cocoa powder, including its ability to fight wrinkles and several other signs of aging. Antioxidants combat the factors that contribute to the aging of your skin. The combination of magnesium and vitamin C in cocoa powder instantly brightens and protects the skin. Cocoa powder also contains omega-6 fats, which speed up the skin's healing process.

CONCLUSION

Now you know how to make different skincare products for your dry skin using natural ingredients, which means you can completely banish toxic ingredients from your skincare routine!

By making these recipes yourself, you know exactly what you're putting on your skin. It is the sure-fire way to ensure your dry skin is treated with only the best ingredients. And the best thing is you'll get that healthy glow, banish those dry patches, and pamper yourself at a fraction of the cost!

You also get some "me-time" since making your own products is, indeed, therapeutic!

I've been using these recipes for quite a while now and my skin has improved a lot. I have noticed a difference in the texture of my skin, and it feels much smoother. My skin is glowing more and is healthier than it has ever been.

I hope the recipes in this book will help your dry skin, too!

With love,

Kinnari Ashar

THANKS FOR READING

Dear reader,

Thank you for reading *How to Heal Dry Skin Naturally*.

If you enjoyed this book, please leave a review where you bought it. It helps more than most people think.

Don't forget your FREE book!

You will also be among the first to know of FREE review copies, discount offers, bonus content, and more.

Go to:

www.SFNonfictionBooks.com/Free-Book

Thanks again for your support.

REFERENCES

100% PURE. (2022, February 1). 6 Reasons to Use Lavender Oil for Skin. 100% PURE. https://www.100percentpure.com/blogs/feed/6-reasons-to-use-lavender-oil-for-skin

Adkins, J., & Hanson, C. (2022, August 26). The Benefits of Cocoa Butter for Your Skin. Byrdie. https://www.byrdie.com/the-benefits-of-cocoa-butter-for-your-skin-3013590

American Academy of Dermatology Association. (n.d.). Dry skin: Who gets and causes. Www.aad.org. https://www.aad.org/public/diseases/a-z/dry-skin-causes

Andrea Jordan. (2021, September 30). Your Dry Skin Patches May Be A Sign Of Another Skin Issue. Women's Health. https://www.womenshealthmag.com/beauty/a19994082/dry-skin-patches-on-face/

Axe, J. (2018, July 30). 10 Proven Myrrh Oil Benefits & Uses. Dr. Axe. https://draxe.com/essential-oils/myrrh-oil/

Baraka Impact. (2022, May 30). Cocoa Powder - Incredible Benefits for your Skin - Baraka Impact. Barakasheabutter.com. https://barakasheabutter.com/blogs/baraka-blogs/cocoa-powder-benefits-for-your-skin

Bella Vita Organic. (2022, March 1). 2022 Magical Benefits of Cucumber for Skin, Face & Body. Bella Vita Organic. https://bellavitaorganic.com/blogs/bellavita-blogs/magical-benefits-of-cucumber-in-2022

Black, T. (2014, June 12). DIY Face Wash. Don't Mess with Mama. https://dontmesswithmama.com/diy-face-wash-facial-cleanser/

Botanical Republic. (2020, March 18). What is Myrrh Oil Used for in Skincare? Botanical Republic. https://www.botanicalrepublic.com/blogs/beauty/what-is-myrrh-oil-used-for-in-skincare

Bovik, N. (2019, October 23). Advantages And Disadvantages Of Having Dry Skin. Sooper Articles. https://www.sooperarticles.com/health-fitness-articles/skin-care-articles/advantages-disadvantages-having-dry-skin-1747793.html

Brady, K. (2019, February 22). How Witch Hazel Can Shrink Your Pores, Absorb Oil, and Give You Younger-Looking Skin. Prevention. https://www.prevention.com/beauty/skin-care/a26450242/witch-hazel-skin-benefits/

Bridger, D. (2019, May 29). DIY Toner: How to Make One for Dry Skin, Oily Skin, Acne and More. Derm Collective. https://dermcollective.com/diy-toner/

Buckler's Team. (2017, January 23). 10 Sweet Almond Oil Benefits for Skin and Hair. Nectar Bath Treats. https://nectarusa.com/blogs/news/10-sweet-almond-oil-benefits-for-skin-and-hair

Chadwick, M. R. (2022, August 23). Marula Oil Is the Hydrating, Anti-inflammatory Solution Derms Love—Here's Why. Byrdie. https://www.byrdie.com/marula-oil-for-skin-4842342

Chakraborty, A. (2022, March 7). 9 Incredible Cucumber Benefits for Skin ~ Study Backed. Bodywise. https://bebodywise.com/blog/cucumber-benefits-for-skin/

Christiansen, S. (2022, January 5). Causes of Dry Patches on Your Face and How to Treat Them. Verywell Health. https://www.verywellhealth.com/dry-patches-on-face-5183942

Conte, A., & Herwitz, K. (2021, November 13). 11 Cheap DIY Face Masks That Let You Have a Spa Day At Home. Woman's Day. https://www.womansday.com/style/beauty/advice/a5005/8-do-it-yourself-home-facials-106030/

Dalela, S. (2021, March 19). How To Use Lavender Essential Oil For Beauty & Aromatherapy. Kama Ayurveda. https://www.kamaayurveda.com/blog/lavender-essential-oil

Dancer, R. (2020, March 13). Five Dry Skin Myths—Busted. Youth to the People. https://www.youthtothepeople.com/blogs/to-the-people/five-dry-skin-myths-busted

Day, G. (2022a, February 15). A 5-Step Morning Skincare Routine For Dry Skin. Beauty Bay Edited. https://www.beautybay.com/edited/morning-skincare-routine-dry-skin/

Day, G. (2022b, February 15). A 6-Step Evening Skincare Routine For Dry Skin. Beauty Bay Edited. https://www.beautybay.com/edited/evening-skincare-routine-dry-skin/

Dweck, C. (2021, April 23). 10 Ways Marula Oil Can Save Your Skin. TheThirty. https://thethirty.whowhatwear.com/marula-oil-benefits

Ecco Verde. (n.d.). 5 Myths About Dry Skin. Ecco Verde Online Shop. Retrieved July 28, 2022, from https://www.ecco-verde.com/info/beauty-blog/5-myths-about-dry-skin

Eucerin. (n.d.). Dry skin on face | Dry skin patches | Eucerin. Www.eucerin.co.uk. https://www.eucerin.co.uk/skin-concerns/dry-skin/dry-and-verydry-facial-skin

Garcia, A. (2019, November 15). 10 Sweet Almond Oil Benefits for Skin and Hair. Nectar Bath Treats. https://nectarusa.com/blogs/news/10-sweet-almond-oil-benefits-for-skin-and-hair

Gerber, S. (2020a, July 20). Homemade Honey Face Wash | Hello-Glow.co. Hello Glow. https://helloglow.co/homemade-honey-face-wash/

Gerber, S. (2020b, November 23). Homemade Face Scrubs for Every Skin Type. Hello Glow. https://helloglow.co/homemade-face-scrubs-every-skin-type/

Gerber, S. (2021, June 24). 6 Ways to Use Rose Essential Oil for Skin. Hello Glow. https://helloglow.co/beauty-ingredient-rose-oil/

Goldenberg Dermatology. (2016, January 7). Common Misconceptions About Dry Skin | Goldenberg Dermatology. Goldenberg

Dermatology. https://goldenbergdermatology.com/blog/common-misconceptions-about-dry-skin/

Grove Collaborative. (2021, July 19). The Ideal Skincare Routine For Dry Skin. Www.grove.co. https://www.grove.co/blog/dry-skin care-routine

Gupta, S. (2020, November 14). Glowing, soft, and radiant skin: That's what apricot oil can do for you. Healthshots. https://www.healthshots.com/beauty/skin-care/4-benefits-of-using-apricot-oil-for-skin/

Gya Labs. (n.d.). Rosemary Essential Oil Benefits & Uses for Skin, Hair & Aromatherapy. Gyalabs.com. Retrieved August 29, 2022, from https://gyalabs.com/pages/guide-rosemary-oil-uses-benefits-skin-hair

Ha, A. (2016, April 13). 5 Myths About Dry Skin. The Singapore Women's Weekly. https://www.womensweekly.com.sg/beauty-and-health/5-myths-about-dry-skin/

Harju, D. (2020, August 31). 3 DIY Facial Cleansers for Dry, Oily + Mature Skin | HelloGlow.co. Hello Glow. https://helloglow.co/3-diy-facial-cleansers-for-dry-oily-mature-skin/

Healthline. (n.d.). How to Exfoliate Safely by Skin Type. Healthline. https://www.healthline.com/health/how-to-exfoliate#how-to

Herbal Dynamics Beauty. (2018, January 25). Cocoa Benefits for Skin: Chocolate Isn't Just for Dessert. Herbal Dynamics Beauty. https://www.herbaldynamicsbeauty.com/blogs/herbal-dynamics-beauty/cocoa-benefits-for-skin-chocolate-isn-t-just-for-dessert

Herd, R. (2017, August 28). 5 Ways Olive Oil Benefits Your Skin. Dermstore. https://www.dermstore.com/blog/olive-oil-benefits-for-skin/

Howard, M. (2020, October 27). Witch Hazel Is Not Your Enemy! 11 Reasons It Belongs In Your Skincare Routine. Women's Health. https://www.womenshealthmag.com/beauty/a19950011/witch-hazel-beauty-benefits/

Hubbard, A., & Timmons, J. (2021, April 29). The Ultimate Skin Care Routine for Dry Skin. Healthline. https://www.healthline.com/health/beauty-skin-care/skin-care-routine-for-dry-skin

JUARA Skincare. (2021, August 17). 5 Benefits Of Avocado Oil For Face & Skin 2022. JUARA Skincare. https://www.juaraskincare.com/blogs/juara-blog/avocado-oil-for-skin

Kakar, P. (2022, January 28). Vitamin E Oil - How To Use It On Your Face, Benefits and Precautions. SkinKraft. https://skinkraft.com/blogs/articles/vitamin-e-oil-for-face

Kashyap, T. (2021a, April 15). 5 Amazing Benefits Of Argan Oil For Beautiful, Glowing Skin. Swirlster.ndtv.com. https://swirlster.ndtv.com/beauty/5-amazing-benefits-of-argan-oil-for-beautiful-glowing-skin-2414104

Kashyap, T. (2021b, June 7). Beauty Benefits Of Carrot Seed Oil For Skincare: How To Use, DIY Remedies. Swirlster.ndtv.com. https://swirlster.ndtv.com/beauty/beauty-benefits-of-carrot-seed-oil-for-skincare-how-to-use-diy-remedies-2458119

Kiehl's. (n.d.). Discover The Benefits of Avocado For Skin | Kiehl's. Kiehl's – Naturally Inspired Skin Care, Body and Haircare. Retrieved September 7, 2022, from https://www.kiehls.com/skin care-advice/avocado-skin-benefits.html

Kilikita, J. (2019, June 20). 7 Spa-Worthy DIY Face Mask Recipes You Can Make At Home. ELLE. https://www.elle.com/uk/beauty/skin/articles/a38190/homemade-diy-face-mask-recipes/

Kluner, E. (n.d.). Home Scrub for Acne. LEAFtv. Retrieved September 6, 2022, from https://www.leaf.tv/4152338/home-scrub-for-acne/

Koganti, S. (2015, April 23). 7 Promising Benefits Of Marula Oil For Skin And Hair. STYLECRAZE. https://www.stylecraze.com/articles/benefits-of-marula-oil/#what-are-the-benefits-of-marula-oil

Laura. (2019, January 8). 5 DIY Face Wash Recipes for All Skin Types. Our Oily House. https://www.ouroilyhouse.com/5-diy-face-wash-recipes-for-all-skin-types/

Laura. (2020a, February 4). 5 Anti-Aging Serum Recipes. Our Oily House. https://www.ouroilyhouse.com/5-anti-aging-serum-recipes/

Laura. (2020b, November 3). DIY Facial Toner with Natural Ingredients. Our Oily House. https://www.ouroilyhouse.com/diy-facial-toner/

Laura. (2022, August 19). Whipped Lavender Sugar Scrub. Our Oily House. https://www.ouroilyhouse.com/homemade-whipped-sugar-scrub/

Leonard, J. (2018, March 18). 4 olive oil benefits for your face. Www.medicalnewstoday.com. https://www.medicalnewstoday.com/articles/321246

Levenberg, C. (2020, September 11). 15 Uses and Benefits of Frankincense Essential Oil. ILAVAHEMP. https://ilavahemp.com/frankincense-essential-oil/#:~:text=Frankincense%20oil%20is%20a%20natural

Life-n-Reflection. (2021, November 3). Homemade Face Serum for Dry Skin That Works Quickly. Life-n-Reflection. https://www.lifenreflection.com/homemade-face-serum-for-dry-skin/

Lifestyle By PS. (2020, June 25). 5 Amazing Benefits Of Using Brown Sugar For Skin – LIFESTYLE BY PS. Lifestylebyps.com. https://lifestylebyps.com/blogs/lifestyle/5-amazing-benefits-of-using-brown-sugar-for-skin

McCabes Pharmacy. (n.d.). Why use Face Masks for Dry Skin? | Routine & Product Advice. Www.mccabespharmacy.com. Retrieved August 1, 2022, from https://www.mccabespharmacy.com/advice-centre/skin-care/face-mask/dry-skin

Menghani, T. (2022, July 14). Apple Cider Vinegar Benefits for Skin | Mamaearth Blog. Mamaearth; Honasa Consumers Pvt. Ltd.

https://mamaearth.in/blog/benefits-of-apple-cider-vinegar-for-skin/

Metzger, C. (2017, September 18). Okay, You Really Need to Be Using Argan Oil on Your Face. Marie Claire; Marie Claire. https://www.marieclaire.com/beauty/news/a17569/argan-oil-for-face/

Moorhouse, V., & Lukas, E. (2022, May 26). How to Exfoliate Your Dry Skin Without Overdoing It. InStyle. https://www.instyle.com/beauty/how-to-exfoliate-dry-skin

Mukherjee, M. (2013, October 24). Brown sugar for healthy, radiant skin - Times of India. The Times of India. https://timesofindia.indiatimes.com/life-style/beauty/brown-sugar-for-healthy-radiant-skin/articleshow/23296908.cms#:~:text=Brown%20sugar

MyGlamm. (n.d.). 5 Benefits of Cocoa Powder for Skin for 2022 - MyGlamm. Www.myglamm.com. Retrieved September 7, 2022, from https://www.myglamm.com/glammstudio/cocoa-powder-benefits-for-skin

Nandi, S. (n.d.). Best Skin Care Routine for Dry Skin. Www.nykaa.com. https://www.nykaa.com/beauty-blog/best-skin-care-routine-for-dry-skin/

Nast, C. (2019, September 19). 10 great ways to use olive oil in your beauty routine that you probably don't know about. Vogue India. https://www.vogue.in/beauty/content/benefits-of-olive-oil-how-to-use-tips-for-skin-care-hair-care

Nordstrom. (2022). The Best Skin Care For Dry Skin. Nordstrom.com. https://www.nordstrom.com/browse/content/blog/dry-skin-routine

Noronha, E. (2020, October 22). Home Remedies For Dry Skin. Femina.in. https://www.femina.in/beauty/skin/home-remedies-for-dry-skin-174433.html

Nourished Essentials. (n.d.). A How-to Guide to Building Your Perfect Homemade Serum for Face. Nourished Essentials. Retrieved August 23, 2022, from https://nourishedessentials.com/blogs/

home/how-to-guide-to-building-your-perfect-homemade-serum-for-face

Pereira, D. (2016, December 15). 5 Benefits Of Cocoa Butter For Your Skin. Be Beautiful India. https://www.bebeautiful.in/all-things-skin/everyday/5-benefits-of-cocoa-butter-for-your-skin

PharmEasy. (2022, March 10). How Does Vitamin E Oil Benefits Your Skin? - PharmEasy. PharmEasy Blog. https://pharmeasy.in/blog/benefits-of-vitamin-e-oil-for-skin/

Poko CBD. (2022, April 3). Apricot Oil for Skin: 15 Benefits of Apricot Oil for Your Skin – Poko CBD. Www.pokocbd.co.uk. https://www.pokocbd.co.uk/blogs/beauty/benefits-of-apricot-oil-for-skin

Pollard, S. (2021, January 11). Make This Aloe Vera Face Wash + Stop Drying Out Your Skin. Hello Glow. https://helloglow.co/aloe-vera-face-wash/

Ready, E. (2022, January 7). Beeswax In Skincare. Bee Cosmetics. https://www.beecosmetics.co.uk/post/beeswax-skincare-benefits

REN Clean Skincare. (2021, January 13). A Complete Skincare Routine for Dry Skin. REN Clean Skincare. https://usa.renskincare.com/blogs/clean-thoughts/a-complete-skincare-routine-for-dry-skin

Robin, M. (2021, October 20). The Unbeatable Benefits of Argan Oil for Your Skin and Hair. Allure. https://www.allure.com/story/argan-oil-benefits-skin-hair

Rodriguez, B., & Hall, C. (2021, July 13). Homemade Face Mask Recipes for Skin That Glows. Marie Claire. https://www.marieclaire.com/beauty/how-to/a2830/best-homemade-face-masks/

Salunkhe, S. (2022, May 30). 5 Skincare Myths You Should Stop Believing, According To Skin Experts. Grazia.co.in. https://www.grazia.co.in/beauty/5-skincare-myths-you-should-stop-believing-according-to-skin-experts-9525.html

Sehgal, K. (2021a, June 1). Olive Oil For Dry Skin: Benefits Of Olive Oil To Get Moisturised And Healthy Skin. Swirlster.ndtv.com. https://swirlster.ndtv.com/beauty/olive-oil-for-dry-skin-benefits-of-olive-oil-to-get-moisturised-and-healthy-skin-2453820

Sehgal, K. (2021b, September 1). 5 Beauty Benefits Of Avocado To Deeply Moisturise And Nourish Dry Skin. Swirlster.ndtv.com. https://swirlster.ndtv.com/beauty/5-beauty-benefits-of-avocado-to-deeply-moisturise-and-nourish-dry-skin-2526192

Sengupta, S. (2018, December 12). Avocado For Skin: How To Use The Superfood To Get Smooth, Young and Glowing Skin. NDTV Food. https://food.ndtv.com/food-drinks/avocado-for-skin-how-to-use-the-superfood-to-get-smooth-young-and-glowing-skin-1961392

Shah, N. (2021, October 25). Amazing Carrot Oil Benefits For Skin And How To Use On Face? Be Beautiful India. https://www.bebeautiful.in/all-things-skin/everyday/carrot-oil-benefits-for-skin#carrot-seed-oil-benefits-for-skin

Shunatona, B. (2022, January 14). Rosehip Oil: How to Use It for Skin Benefits and the Best Products to Try. Cosmopolitan. https://www.cosmopolitan.com/style-beauty/beauty/a38741835/rosehip-oil-benefits/

Sinha, R. (2013, November 21). Best Skin Care Routine For Dry Skin – Daily Skin Care Routine To Follow At Home. Stylecraze. https://www.stylecraze.com/articles/daily-routine-for-dry-skin/

Sinha, R. (2021, March 2). 5 Benefits Of Avocado Oil For Skin, How To Use, And Warnings. STYLECRAZE. https://www.stylecraze.com/articles/avocado-oil-for-skin/

Skin Functional. (2022, March 2). Common Myths About Dry Skin | SKIN functional. Https://Skinfunctional.com/. https://skinfunctional.com/dry-skin-myths-you-should-stop-believing/

Spruch-Feiner, S. (2021, August 19). Everything You Need to Know About Using Argan Oil for Smooth Skin. Byrdie. https://www.byrdie.com/argan-oil-for-skin-5080152

Suhale, S. (2021, April 8). 12 Homemade Natural Toners for Dull and Dry Skin You Should Definitely Give a Try. Optimistic Girls. https://optimisticgirls.com/homemade-natural-toners/

Suvarna. (2020, October 5). 10 Excellent DIY Homemade Moisturizers for Dry Skin!! Styles at Life. https://stylesatlife.com/articles/home-made-moisturizers-for-dry-skin/

Tadimalla, R. T. (2014, November 5). 11 Rosehip Oil Benefits, Possible Side Effects, & How To Use It. STYLECRAZE. https://www.stylecraze.com/articles/amazing-benefits-of-rose-hip-oil/

Team TC46. (2020, October 27). 9 Homemade Moisturizers To Treat Dull & Dry Skin. The Channel 46. https://www.thechannel46.com/beauty/skin-care/prevent-dry-skin-this-autumn-winter-with-9-easy-to-make-diy-moisturizer-recipes/

UPMC HealthBeat. (2018, April 3). Do You Have Dry, Flaky Skin on Your Face? Here's What You Can Do. UPMC HealthBeat. https://share.upmc.com/2018/04/dry-flaky-skin-on-face/

Vartan, S. (2021, November 8). 8 Recipes for Homemade Natural Moisturizers for Face and Body. Treehugger. https://www.treehugger.com/natural-moisturizer-5194041

Veda Oils. (n.d.). DIY Homemade Cleanser for Dry Skin - Benefits & How to Use. VedaOils. Retrieved August 4, 2022, from https://www.vedaoils.com/blogs/news/homemade-cleanser-for-dry-skin

Visagenics Premium Essential Oils. (n.d.). [2022] Benefits & Uses of Rose Oil for Skin | Full Guide. Visagenics Premium Essential Oils. https://www.visagenics.com/blogs/blog/2020-benefits-of-rose-oil-for-skin

Vora, D. (2022, February 24). The 101 Of Maintaining Dry Skin. MyCocoSoul. https://mycocosoul.com/blogs/skin-care-regimen/skincare-routine-for-dry-skin

Vyas, S. (2020, July 14). 10 Easy DIY Face Masks To Treat Your Dry Skin | by Smriti Vyas. Sociomix. https://www.sociomix.com/

diaries/beauty/10-easy-diy-face-masks-to-treat-your-dry-skin/
1594739736

Walden, H. (2019, September 24). Face Mask for Dry Skin: Benefits, Home Remedies and How To Pick One. Derm Collective. https:// dermcollective.com/face-mask-for-dry-skin/

Wnek, D. (2022, March 15). Is Witch Hazel Actually Good for Your Skin? Good Housekeeping. https://www.goodhousekeeping.com/ beauty-products/a38488805/witch-hazel-skin-benefits/

Image References

About time. (2019). Human skin layers, healthcare and medical illustration about human skin [Online image]. In iStock. https:// www.istockphoto.com/vector/human-skin-layers-gm1149397551-310741858?phrase=layers%20of%20skin

Bezrodny, A. (2017). Chart ph alkaline and acidic scale vector illustration [Online image]. In iStock. https://www.istockphoto.com/ vector/chart-ph-alkaline-and-acidic-scale-vector-gm817607620-132311597?phrase=ph%20scale

natianis. (2019). Basic skin condition type chart, normal, dry, sensitive, combination, oily, acne prone. Line vector illustration, design template. [Online image]. In iStock. https://www.istockphoto.com/ vector/basic-skin-types-chart-line-vector-illustration-gm1166107402-321092217?phrase=skin%20types%20face

AUTHOR RECOMMENDATIONS

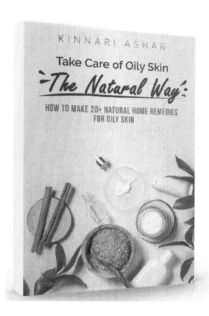

Discover How to Stop Oily Skin... For Good!

Make your own all-natural products today, because everyone deserves clean and clear skin.

Get it now.

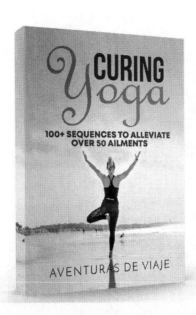

Discover How to Use Yoga as Medicine

Get your hands on *Curing Yoga*, because with it you can heal your mind, body, and spirit.

Get it now.

www.SFNonfictionBooks.com/Free-Book

ABOUT KINNARI

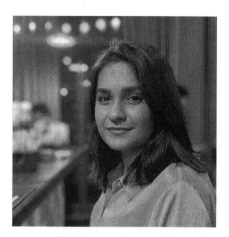

Kinnari Ashar has been passionate about beauty and lifestyle since her early teens. Ever since, she has sought out knowledge, techniques, skills, and trends in the niche.

Though a Biomedical Engineer by formal education, she chose to carve a path for herself as a writer, a blogger, and an influencer through constant learning, experimentation, and knowledge sharing.

www.SFNonfictionBooks.com

amazon.com/kinnari-ashar/e/B0BGH6762F

goodreads.com/KinnariAshar

facebook.com/glowinmist

instagram.com/kinnari.ashar

Made in the USA
Middletown, DE
21 May 2024